MARIJUANA:

Guide To Illness And Pain Management

3rd Edition

by Mary Soloman

The trademarks that are used are without any consent, and the publication of the trademark is without permission or backing by the trademark owner. All trademarks and brands within this book are for clarifying purposes only and are owned by the owners themselves, not affiliated with this document.

TABLE OF CONTENTS

INTRODUCTION

If you are like many of Americans, you or your loved ones suffer from chronic pain. Cancer, arthritis, back injuries, migraines, nerve damage, autoimmune diseases and many other causes of pain debilitate millions of people every day. Many feel trapped in an endless cycle of taking addictive pain medication in order to function in their daily lives. Having an alternative to all of these chemically produced medicines has given the rise for hope in states where the legality of marijuana use has been accepted, either for medical or for recreational use.

Medical marijuana is slowly becoming available throughout the country. Pain relief is the most well recognized and studied effect of marijuana. Unfortunately, there continues to be a great deal of innocent confusion surrounding the medication, leaving many American's under treated. Myths, most of which have been debunked by scientific research, continue to be spread throughout the mainstream media. However, what is clear from users is that the benefits derived from the use of marijuana are worthwhile and make the pain seemingly less hard to bear.

This book will help you determine if medical marijuana is for you

If you have already decided medical marijuana would be a good treatment for you but are unsure about how to use the drug, or which strains to use for the illness you have, this book is for you as it gives you clear indications of cases in which medical marijuana has proven to be useful and beneficial.

This book seeks to address some of the myths and offer compelling information on how these are just myths and not based on fact. You will also get information on whether or not medical grade marijuana is the right treatment for you and how to go about purchasing it or getting a prescription for marijuana based ready prepared medications. You will also get familiar with how medical marijuana compares to pain medications, the different ways you can use medical marijuana, what symptoms it can treat, and how it relieves pain.

The purpose of this book is to give an unbiased opinion. While there are many myths about the negative sides of marijuana, which can be far-fetched, the herb still has some side effects. These are also covered in detail as well as giving tips to potential growers who wish to supply their own needs.

I hope that with the help of this book you will build your own opinion about whether or not marijuana is for you and that, in the process, you will learn about a very old botanical plant that has an extremely long history of helping people with medical ailments. It's hard to believe that people are still arguing the case for use of marijuana when it has been in use since before the days of Christ. That makes a pretty powerful statement as to people's belief in the healing powers that it has. Read on, and enjoy your journey into the story of marijuana and its use worldwide, for therapeutic and for recreational purposes.

This book may also be useful to share with parents or for parents using marijuana medically to share with children, so that a clearer understanding can be gleaned of how marijuana has the potential to help the sick. That deeper understanding can open up doors to building very strong relationships and there is no content within the book that is unsuitable to younger readers. All contents have been written to try to help readers to understand a little more about a topic that may have been "controversial" until recently even if you live in a state that now accepts that marijuana use for medical reasons is justified. Being open minded to the possibility that marijuana may help those suffering will help you to support them in their hour of need. For those considering taking medical marijuana, it may also be useful to share this book with people who are close to you, so that they can understand why you have chosen this path.

Acceptance of Marijuana as Being Helpful

It has been a very long road for those fighting for the right to use Marijuana for medical reasons, even though history has shown that marijuana has been used for so long for the properties it has against certain medical conditions. If you look through the history of the use of marijuana, it would appear that use of this wonder plant go way back and that it was even used BC because of its ability to help people with illnesses.

One may be surprised to learn that in 1980, tests were performed to see if smoked marijuana had better results than pharmaceutical drugs that imitated the active THC that has been found to be the part of the marijuana that helps those who need it. These tests were done by the National Cancer Institute and found that the anti-vomiting drug, Marinol, was not as effective. Regardless of this, one can only assume that the profits the pharmaceutical companies stood to lose if marijuana was introduced as a legal alternative were considered too much. Following these trials that showed a definite improvement in patients who smoked marijuana, no other really convincing argument could be made. The shame is that patients' care was less important than the actual sales of pharmaceutical drugs and the idea of cannabis use was dismissed and made illegal.

There have been various studies throughout the years that proved the beneficial effects of cannabis, though the

1980 study was to prove a turning point. The following year, Alice O'Leary and Bob Randall formed an association to help people that needed marijuana for medical purposes to gain access to it, via the legal battles that followed. This was an alliance that helped patients to obtain the right to use marijuana for medical reasons.

The precedent had already been set in November 1976 by a man who was suffering from glaucoma and who stated that he had no choice other than to use marijuana to retain his quality of life. The ruling by Judge James Washington, allowed Robert Randall to continue to use marijuana for the treatment of what was indeed a medical disorder. Thus, the association formed to help people obtain marijuana for medical reasons was run by people who had already been through the loopholes and knew how to gain positive results.

The map shown below shows the states that have now accepted that marijuana can be used for medicinal purposes, although some states have gone so far as to accept that it can also be used for recreational purposes.

Meanwhile countries across the globe are at odds with whether marijuana can be accepted as an aid in the case of people whose illnesses merit it. In the United Kingdom, there is no provision for this being acceptable, although tolerance levels for small amounts of marijuana for personal use seems to be the order of the day. In France, Sativex, which is spray using marijuana as its base was approved last year. In reality, though, this doesn't guarantee that it will be released and no news has been heard yet as to when this will become available. There is no tolerance to marijuana use in France and thus it is thought that it will be a very long time before the medical profession and lawmakers will really recognize its therapeutic uses.

Holland is one country that was pivotal in the free use of marijuana, although have experienced problems since tourists flocked there to smoke it in cafes in the capital with the intention of taking large quantities home. Thus, limitations had to be placed on non-locals so that Holland could not be blamed for breaches of the law in other countries, when visitors went home.

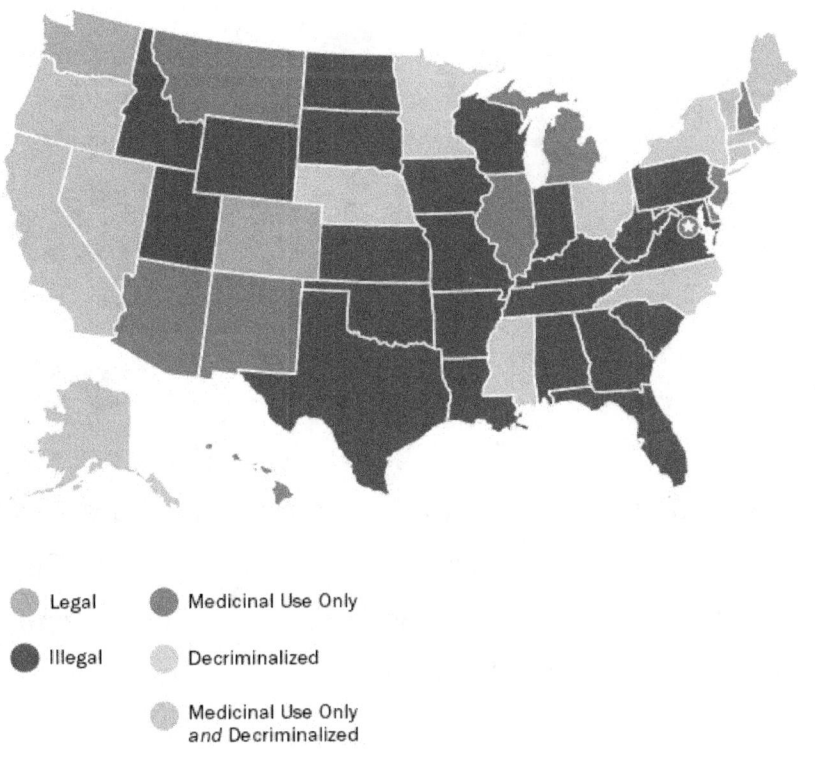

Legal

Medicinal Use Only

Illegal

Decriminalized

Medicinal Use Only
and Decriminalized

Marijuana has always been used in Moroccan society and is considered a norm to take with mint tea, although even here, what appeared to be happening was that vendors would sell poor quality cannabis to tourists.

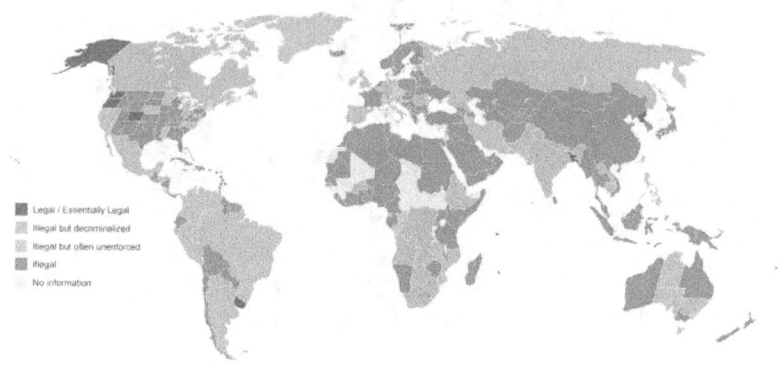

As you can see from the above map, there are very few places in the world where marijuana use is legal. The blue areas represent this. A far greater proportion of countries still consider the use of marijuana as illegal and that includes for medical use.

Interestingly enough Uruguay has stated that marijuana use is not illegal in their country, although the change to the law to reinforce this has been delayed until 2015 and will be interesting to follow.

CHAPTER ONE

MEDICAL USE OF MARIJUANA

As well as the States shown on the map at the beginning of this chapter, certain countries have accepted medical use of marijuana as being legal. Spain, Finland, Portugal and more recently Germany has been looking into the potential of allowing this use. This seems to be a pattern in that much investigation is being done in many of the countries that consider marijuana as an illegal substance, though little seems to have been achieved in those countries to help in the acceptance of the usefulness of the drug. In the meantime, people who are suffering from MS and many serious conditions are being deprived of the law backing their use of marijuana to give them relief from the illnesses suffered. The fight within those countries continues.

It's vital to read the history of the use of marijuana to get a fuller picture of how its use is backed up by history, but in fact has been discouraged in the last century in favor of pharmaceutical drugs. Both can be useful and the history section of this book shows you the established record of how marijuana has been used since as far back as BC. Thus, it's unsure why people are so opposed to it becoming a norm for people with illnesses that cause symptoms that can be improved with marijuana use.

Another interesting contrast is that alcohol, which is known to cause serious liver problems and smoking commercially produced cigarettes which is known to cause cancer are both seen as acceptable behaviors. One can only assume that governments who encourage the use of either would miss the revenue from these.

In that light, would it not therefore be beneficial for countries not yet accepting medical use of marijuana to look into the potential revenue that could be made from its legalization. In countries where there is no allowance for medical use, unfortunately, the cost of marijuana is dictated by dealers who are renowned to want vast profits to cover the risk that they take moving marijuana from one country to another.

With a general acceptance that marijuana can be of help to the sick, it would seem unreasonable if countries were not even prepared to investigate the potential of medicines which contain it and the potential of growing profitable crops from which each government could gain reasonable revenue from taxes.

The use of marijuana for medical purposes is longstanding. It's not something new or invented by the young simply so that they can keep up with trends followed by peers. Yes, THC can give kids a high, but used for what it is intended, this can be a very powerful aid to people who are suffering. If you think of it in that light, there are other things which kids may put to uses not intended such as glue, used in sniffing, alcohol used without the caution adults may use and this book is really about serious users of marijuana for medical use, rather than for recreational purposes.

CHAPTER TWO

THE HISTORY OF THE USE OF MARIJANA

The use of marijuana for treating medical ailments goes back beyond the time of Jesus. In fact, it's first recorded use shows that in 2900 BC, it was used as a yin yan medicine by the Chinese under Emperor Fu Hsi and this use has been tracked by a book entitled "Hemp: The Plant with a Divided History."

The National Institute of Drug Abuse, during research that took place in the 1970s stated that medical marijuana predates all recorded history but that its use in 1500 BC can be established. Thus, one can see that cannabis has long been recognized as having healing powers, and this wasn't just guesswork. Although they didn't have the research facilities that are available today, the work that went on with what little they did have showed practical use of marijuana had positive results and that should be pretty convincing to skeptics.

In Egypt, one use of cannabis that was very consistent with later findings early in the last century was that it helped people with glaucoma. The National Eye Institute and the Institute of Medicine argue that there is little evidence that there was an improvement or that cannabis lowered the recovery rate of people with glaucoma, although earlier suggestions stated that marijuana was used to lower the pressure on the eye and that IOP (or pressure) could be lowered up to three to four hours, by using marijuana either smoked or if administered orally, such as in food. The jury is out on this since the study also revealed that smoking of marijuana could actually increase the rate at which the heart was beating and decrease blood pressure. Topical creams containing marijuana were not included in this study or considered as viable.

One thing that is sure is that marijuana had enough power to be used in a mixture with milk as an anesthetic as far back as 1000 BC. Around the same time, it was used for ailments that included a wide variety of ailments. In fact, people in India had strong beliefs that marijuana helped to quicken the mind and thought the importance of marijuana as a medicinal plant had great importance. They even believed that it had the potential to cure leprosy.

In the year 1 AD, written records were kept in China listing marijuana in a recipe book where it was recommended for medical use, after being dried out. The value of the plant was that it could be used for so many ailments and amusingly enough included the ailment of absentmindedness.

There is a very good historical background of marijuana shown **here** which backs up that marijuana has been considered suitable for many different ailments over such a long period of time that questioning its use may seem a little unreasonable. Many of the herbs used in times when there were no real pharmaceutical cures are still used in complementary medicine to this date.

Looking back through records kept on the use of marijuana, some things become a little less easy to understand. For example, while marijuana is said to relax patients and make them less aware of pain and able to avoid some of the side effects of serious cancer treatments, many countries still refuse to allow its use, even though those who do are giving their residents the freedom of choice.

In the United States of America, the first state to actually outlaw the use of cannabis was in fact Massachusetts although, in fairness to the government of that time, they did try to tackle many social problems including the consumption of alcohol, gambling, oral sex and prizefighting. That's quite a lot of things to prohibit in one sitting, though it seems that the prohibition of cannabis was more to stop it becoming a problem, rather than being due to a belief that cannabis actually did any harm.

Prohibition dealt with current society problems but it also dealt with potential problems. This way of thinking though has little place in a society that have laws which cover responsible use of those items which were previously prohibited. The biggest hurdle that marijuana has had to face is because of negative connections brought about by only seeing marijuana as a way to get "high" as opposed to being a real way forward in helping sick people deal with pain and suffering.

CHAPTER THREE

WHAT IS MEDICAL GRADE MARIJUANA

Medical marijuana simply refers to use of cannabis for herbal therapy as recommended by a physician. Marijuana is actually dried cannabis, and its narcotic effect is mainly due to the substance THC, whose content varies between 0.2% and 20% depending on the type of cannabis farming method and other associated factors, as explained within this book.

Smoking medical grade marijuana can actually be good for you. It has been quite helpful in assisting people suffering from cancer, glaucoma, migraines, diabetes, rheumatism, multiple sclerosis, anorexia, AIDS, Parkinson's disease, and

Alzheimer's disease. Marijuana also relieves stomach pain and the side effects of chemotherapy, suppresses nausea and vomiting, relieves muscle cramps and treats muscle injuries, helps with loss of appetite, and restlessness.

There are concerns that smoking marijuana causes physical and psychological addiction, weakens the immune system, interferes with reproduction, and may cause cancer. However, no real evidence and confirmed research has proven this. Links to cancer could be made, however, with the use of marijuana in conjunction with tobacco and perhaps people who are against the use of marijuana to support their case may use this link. Those who do use marijuana without using tobacco, however, may still be reaping the benefits of its use. There are others that argue that if you are inhaling anything into your lungs, and then this cannot be good for your health. Although today we are seeing more and more people opting to smoke electronic cigarettes as an alternative to tobacco filled cigarettes, and perhaps they too are breathing something into the lungs that may be discovered in the future. It's perhaps too early to judge this new habit.

One thing that should be borne in mind is that if there are benefits from smoking marijuana, then being without a supply, may cause a psychological need. Simply because those same symptoms for which it was taken may return. Therefore, while not strictly addictive, there is a dependence upon a regular supply. Thus, legalization of marijuana for medical use should take into account the need that the patient has for regularity of supply.

While medical marijuana may be useful in different ways, you will need to determine if it is suitable for you. Consult with your physician to direct you accordingly or talk to a marijuana center who can give you more advice. You may not only need to consult your physician but also a medical marijuana caregiver or physician. They can direct you on how to experiment with cannabis and the different strains in order to determine which strain is best for you. It will be important for you to know some of the marijuana strains available. Read up on what your medical center literature says, as the strains available to you may differ geographically. You will also need to know the cost involved, since medicines of any kind will come with a price tag.

One of the arguments supporters for the legalization of marijuana for medical purposes has used to back up their argument is that in cases where legal use is introduced, the government may actually be able to make money on taxes derived from the supply of marijuana, rather than leaving the profits in the hands of criminals and drug traffickers. This would also mean that people using marijuana for medical or approved recreational purposes would need no contact with dealers of illegal drugs and would thus be less likely to come into contact with those drugs or become involved in their use.

Medical grade marijuana will also mean standardization so if this is applicable in your state, then you don't have to worry about whether the drug supplied is of good quality or not. This is a move toward making treatment with marijuana uniform from state to state which can only be a good thing and help to eliminate profit making by unscrupulous dealers who have no accountability for the quality of the marijuana supplied by them.

Medical grade marijuana is that which contains something called CBD (or cannabidiol). This has been proven to be very effective in cases of patients suffering from schizophrenia and to be useful as an anti-convulsive treatment. CBD may also be interesting from a female perspective, since it is reported to decrease the incidence of breast cancer formation.

People who use cannabis to relieve any medical symptom can class the cannabis that they use as being "medical grade" though with the extended use of pesticides and insecticides may mean that the cannabis chosen is contaminated. Street marijuana also has the added disadvantage because the user does not usually know the history of the plant or exactly where it came from. Little regulation means that it could already be contaminated and that includes being loaded with chemicals to try and avoid detection by trained dogs.

Thus, medical marijuana in the true sense, i.e. produced and supplied by companies approved by the medical authorities, must therefore assist in ensuring that the quality bought is the best possible for the illness that is being treated.

CHAPTER FOUR

MYTHS ABOUT MARIJUANA

The myths surrounding marijuana and its use are quite far-fetched. This chapter seeks to look at some of these myths and the scientific research that discredits the myths. This may make interesting reading if you are a little skeptical about the use of marijuana, bearing in mind the fact that many countries dismiss the plant as a drug to be classed with others that are considered as potentially harmful to the health. This misclassification adds to the confusion of those seeking information on the usefulness of marijuana to help with individual illnesses.

Marijuana is Addictive

This is probably one of the biggest myths about marijuana. Most people actually think that using marijuana is the gateway to the use of other hardcore drugs. While statistics show that people who illegally use marijuana are far more likely to get addicted to other drugs, marijuana does not share any other harmful properties with these drugs.

Marijuana is not addictive, although it is possible to become psychologically dependent on marijuana. Dependency is often because of the pain relief felt from using the drug. Pain relief may be in the form of physical pain or psychological pain such as anxiety or depression but if the marijuana is helping that suffering, then of course, when it is stopped, it will be missed.

It is important to know that medical marijuana and illegally bought marijuana are two different things. While medical marijuana is clean, illegally bought marijuana is often mixed with other substances or chemicals. It could also have been transported by dubious means from country to country meaning that it could have been contaminated en route. A health care provider prescribes medical marijuana. The daily dosage is monitored, just like with any other medication. Thus, the amount prescribed will be the amount that the physician or specialist believes to be suitable for treating the patient's illness or symptoms. It isn't free license to have as much as one wants.

The doctor prescribing the marijuana for a patient will be aware of the patient's records. Just as pharmaceutical drugs can be counterproductive, so can the use of marijuana in conjunction with some anti-depressants. That means that the doctor needs to evaluate the patient need based on his history, his illness and what drugs are currently being prescribed.

Smoking Marijuana can lead to lung cancer:
Cannabis is more damaging to lungs than cigarettes

It is nearly impossible to smoke the same amount of marijuana in a day as someone smoking cigarettes. Actually more people die from smoking cigarettes as compared to those dying from AIDs, car accidents, murders and alcohol combined. Thus, clearly, this belief is in something that is mythical rather than based on any medical evidence.

In 2010, The National Institute on Drug Abuse indicated that marijuana smoke contains some of the same cancer causing compounds as tobacco. However, scientists have yet to find any definitive link between smoking marijuana and increased chances of lung cancer. What should be borne in mind here is that many marijuana smokers choose to mix marijuana with tobacco to make a "joint" and the tobacco element has the same danger as it does in cigarette format.

If the smoker then inhales deeper than he/she would when smoking cigarettes, then the potential danger increases. It is known that marijuana smokers do inhale deeply and perhaps this contributes a little to the notion that marijuana can cause cancer, although there is little research to back this as an indisputable fact.

Marijuana can cure illnesses

No research has actually shown that marijuana can cure anything. Marijuana is mainly known for its palliative effects in dealing with such symptoms as nausea, muscle spasticity and pain. You may wonder if marijuana is truly medicinal, why is it not available in licensed pharmacies. This is usually because doctors argue that they cannot legally prescribe drugs that are said to have no medical benefit.

However, one could argue that many pharmaceutical drugs have very little effect and that some are placebos. There are also medicines available in pharmacies that are produced by homeopathy labs and also natural treatments available in health stores. Doctors may only recommend pot in states where medical marijuana legislation has been passed and where it is generally accepted that marijuana has beneficial use. Dietary supplements also have a worse reputation than marijuana and are often used as a means to adjust poor diet caused by convenience foods whereas the better way would be to take responsibility for the food being eaten and to avoid having to take excessive vitamins and supplements which may be counterproductive when taken with heavy consumption of coffee.

There is no "safe" dosage of marijuana

This statement is quite misleading, considering that scientists have not even found a lethal dose of marijuana. There is no known lethal dose of marijuana. It is estimated that you would actually need to consume 1500 pounds of marijuana in fifteen minutes in order to die. As a contrast, people have joked about dying from marijuana being possible if a ten ton block was to hit you from a great height, though of course, this is tongue in cheek and only used to demonstrate the impossibility of overdose.

Teen use of marijuana increases in medical marijuana states

Most people are of the opinion that legalizing the use of marijuana sends the wrong message to children, implying that it is okay to use marijuana or other drugs. However, recent studies indicate that the availability of medical marijuana doesn't lead to an increase in teen use of marijuana. Recent research undertaken in Rhode Island compared the teen use of pot to that of Massachusetts, which does not have a medical marijuana law, and found that there was no difference in user rates. Since teens are rarely given marijuana as a medical treatment, it is very unlikely that the legalization of marijuana use prescribed by doctors will make any difference whatsoever.

Hemp is the same as Marijuana

Yes, hemp is in the same plant genus as marijuana, but it is not marijuana. Hemp has a relatively low concentration of THC, the main ingredient in pot that usually makes a person feel high. It also has high amounts of cannabidiol that are known to counteract the effect of THC. Thus, you can smoke a very large hemp cigar and not get high.

The only reason hemp is illegal is due to the overall prohibition on cannabis plants. In some countries, though, hemp is used for the production of fabric, ropes and other associated produce as this is very popular with modern day earth conscious people.

The clothing fabric is very hardwearing and many markets use it for both male and female fashion items, as well as handbags and other accessories. Since the level of THC is practically nonexistent, some countries are even tolerant of crops being grown in specific areas for this use and these are controlled to ensure that illegal plants are not grown. Other countries have preferred to ban the growth of all marijuana because that leaves no doubt about whether the plant is of the hemp variety or the variety that produces THC.

Marijuana has no medicinal value

You will be surprised at the many studies that have concluded that marijuana is a valuable herbal therapy for numerous illnesses. These studies indicate that marijuana can relieve pain, nausea and vomiting, can stimulate appetite, fight cancerous tumors, help prevent seizures, relieve muscle spasticity, and many other things. Those that argue against it should be more versed with its history and look into it more thoroughly since this is a narrow view, considering the long term use of marijuana as an aid to health.

Cannabis use leads to apathy and lack of motivation

A study in humans given higher doses of cannabis periodically throughout the day or during the week found that there is no loss of motivation. Of course, regular abuse of pain medications could reduce a person's functionality, but cannabis has not shown to do that. It is a myth that a person using marijuana will turn into a lazy, couch potato. There is a certain leaning toward relaxation and that's quite different from being lazy.

One needs to consider that cannabis use may make someone a little lethargic, though this relaxation may be considered to be therapeutic. People may mistake this for lack of motivation. However, people who do take marijuana may be very creative. There are various medical findings that show that different strains of marijuana give differing levels of creativity and some had very little, though these were hybrid types not commonly used for medical use.

Genetic alteration to certain types of cannabis plants has been experimented with since the 70s though users of natural cannabis argue that cannabis in its natural form is what is healing and helpful to users who need it for medical purposes. Some of the heavier types of cannabis produced via modification seem to give the effect of making people lose some of the creativity gleaned from unaltered crops where the THC levels have not been tampered with. These altered crops tend to make people lethargic and withdrawn which are not desirable effects.

Cannabis use causes memory loss, diminished intelligence and logical thinking

Laboratory tests show that cannabis does reduce short-term memory, but only while under the influence. Since this is limited to several hours, this is not a long term problem. If you look at the effects of alcohol that is an accepted form of stimulation, the alcohol use is far more harmful to logical thinking and causes violence that has never been associated with marijuana use.

There is currently no scientific evidence that marijuana impairs long-term memory but there is a study that shows improved IQ levels in people who smoke regularly but in moderate amounts. The Canadian Medical Association Journal published the study that was performed using people who do not smoke, those who smoke moderate amounts of marijuana and those who were heavy users. The IQ levels of the participants had already been measured during their youth and the amount of marijuana smoked was verified by urine tests.

What was amazing were the findings which were published on Spirit Science and Metaphysics website. Later findings by a US study backed up those results and used 1300 adults. This was performed at the John Hopkins University in Baltimore and showed that light and heavy smokers of marijuana did not experience any more cognitive decline than others within the group who did not smoke.

This was further followed by a study at Harvard that tested people who had smoked marijuana at least 5,000 times during their lifetimes, and that no difference in IQ was present as compared against people who did not smoke. The report further went on to state that irresponsible use of marijuana was not considered in the study and that partying and using marijuana as an escape from school or responsibilities was not what was being studied and of course, should be avoided.

Cannabis use leads to crime

You may have heard the myth that cannabis use causes violence and aggression and consequently leads to crime. Actually, a recent study that was in the journal *PLOS* found that the states legalizing medical marijuana did not experience an increase in crime rates. The crime rates either remained the same or decreased. It is important to note that the reason many countries have banned the use of marijuana is because the majority of users are technically classified as criminals because of possession of drugs, not because of violent crime.

It should further be noted that there is more violence associated with alcohol than there has ever been with cannabis. Whereas cannabis may calm people and make them very peaceful and tranquil, alcohol tends to do the opposite, making people much more aggressive and agitated.

Marijuana is dangerous since it contains over 400 chemicals

How many things do we consume daily that have thousands of chemicals? Singling out marijuana because of high chemical content is simply misleading. Very misleading! Did you know coffee contains 1500 chemicals? It's a very limiting statement indeed and it's worth looking at the larger picture because chemicals contained in actual pharmaceutical medicines are not thought of as a threat to health simply because they are given the label of "medicines." If you were to look into the long term dangers of taking some "medicines" which have been approved by the FDA, then you may see that cannabis is a much more natural product and perhaps has more value than some manufactured drugs.

It's also worth reading some labels in supermarkets and looking how many chemicals you are ingesting every day of the week in your day to day food supplies. With much of these being produced in factories and added shelf life being an incentive to use all kinds of preservatives, you may just be shocked at how many chemicals are contained in the food that you buy.

There's a very interesting article here that will show you exactly what is meant by foods containing chemicals. It's actually very scary what people consume and how much these contain potentially harmful chemicals. Marijuana may have natural chemicals as part of its makeup, though these are useful in the fight against pain.

Current marijuana is far more potent than it was many years ago

There is actually no medical evidence showing that low-potency marijuana is less harmful than high-potency marijuana. Actually, high-potency marijuana is preferable since you will consume less of it to achieve the desired effects, which reduces the amount of smoke entering the lungs. This will lower the risk of getting various respiratory health hazards. Saying that high-potency marijuana is more harmful than low potency marijuana is like saying that wine is more harmful than beer.

What should be taken into account here is the user's experience with that particular strain. This will affect how potent that marijuana will be to the individual. As stated earlier, genetic alteration and hybrid varieties perhaps do give cause for concern, though the natural plant in its various natural varieties is known for its healing properties and that is generally accepted by scientists and doctors all over the world, even though some countries still fight its legalization for medical purposes.

One could wonder whether there is a link between this bad reputation and the amount of money made by pharmaceutical companies who would lose revenue if other countries were to decide to take the same route as many of the states have done, in legalization of cannabis as a relief to medical problems.

There is an interesting side to all of this, because no doubt pharmaceutical companies will gear themselves up to produce cannabis based products, so that they do not miss out on the potential profits. Since pharmaceutical companies tend to think big, it is also worrying to the general smoking population that they may use genetic engineering to produce the quantities that they need to supply the future demand.

At the moment, they are producing cannabis based pharmaceutical medicines that are prescribed by doctors in the states where this is permitted. Dronabinol, Nabilone and Nabiximols are already being produced to meet demand and these are drugs that are classed as pharmaceutical. These come in pill and liquid format and spray format Sativex was approved in January 2014 in France for use in medical treatment for pain relief although this has not yet hit the pharmacies.

There was an article in the newspaper in France that coupled the amount of profit that would be made by pharmaceutical companies and the amount of loss that would be sustained by the government in fines for possession and customs fines. Thus, it's unlikely that Sativex will be allowed to hit the market at any time soon. The story continues.

The point being made here is that indeed the potency of marijuana isn't what has changed, except in GM produced strains. For medical crops that are home grown, this is unlikely to show any change in potency.

CHAPTER FIVE

VARIETIES AND STRAINS OF MARIJUANA

Marijuana strains can be either hybrid varieties or pure breeds of cannabis; Cannabis Sativa or Cannabis Indica. Cannabis Indica strains mostly originate from the strains in Afghanistan, Pakistan, Bangladesh and India where they were mainly used for production of hashish. Smoking indica mainly results in a heavier sedation state resulting in pain relief. Some of these strains include Blueberry, Northern lights, LA confidential, purple kush, Buba Kush, and OG kush.

Cannabis sativa plants are quite different from indica in that they grow quite long and take a longer time to flower. These strains are known for their uplifting properties, making them the best for relieving anxiety, depression, and muscle tension. Some of the common strains are Casey Jones, Blue Dream, Trainwreck, Strawberry cough, sour Diesel, and Purple Haze.

Currently, hybrid marijuana strains are very common. This is mainly because the cross breeding leads to better strains. Some of the common hybrids include White widow, AK-47, Lemon Skunk, Master Kush, Jack Herer, and NYC Diesel.

Although these strains are mentioned in passing, it's merely for reference for those interested in the history and use of marijuana. The strains used for medical marijuana are more likely to give sedative results and a sense of calm, which is useful for people who have MS or pain related illnesses. They are also useful to help counter the side effects of cancer treatment and the exotic names that you see above are unlikely to be associated with medical use.

Many of the plants that are grown for medical use derive from countries where these exotic hybrids are grown, though the basic plant is what will be used in general as a medical aid or treatment.

The more exotic breeds can be heavier in sedation and also make reality harder to grasp. These are not recommended treatments at all, since escape is not the purpose of medical marijuana use. They may also produce negative results such as anti social behavior and withdrawal from company.

The strains that are smuggled into the US for illegal use, as stated previously, may have pollutants in them that should be considered by those who try cannabis. During the trafficking many of these are carried in garbage trucks and can be mixed with unknown chemicals to make the amount look larger and more valuable, in order to try and increase the profits made by drug barrens.

Since medical marijuana use is supervised and clinics are available for help and guidance, then seeking that help is a more sensible way forward than to experiment with drugs which have an unknown history which have been imported illegally.

CHAPTER SIX

HOW TO PURCHASE MARIJUANA

All marijuana can actually be considered medical grade due to its therapeutic effect, except as explained in previous chapters. It is as simple as this: if you are using marijuana to ease or treat a medical condition, you are using marijuana medicinally. As you make a decision to purchase marijuana for medical use, you need to know that marijuana strength varies from one strain to the other. Some strains have as little content of THC as 2% and as much as 30%.

You also have the question of where you are buying it and the background information that may make a difference as to the actual content of the marijuana you are purchasing. If this is in "soap" format, then it's harder to be sure of the exact content of that lump which is weighed and charged for according to weight.

When purchasing medical marijuana, it is advisable to buy marijuana that is organically grown, as it is free from fertilizers and other chemicals. Buying marijuana illegally from some clinics or street dealers can prove to be disastrous since much of the marijuana is likely to be contaminated. Such marijuana may be transported in garbage trucks and wrapped with a number of dangerous chemicals in order to mask the scent to avoid customs. Some unscrupulous dealers may also add lead to marijuana to increase its weight.

It's important to purchase pure marijuana as consuming contaminated marijuana can cause more harm than good. Thus locally grown organic produce is preferable to that which is sold through the black market. If you ask your advice center about where to purchase it, they will have lists of producers who are approved and this gives you the edge.

If you are prescribed the drugs that contain marijuana, then these will of course be available on prescription from a pharmacy and your doctor will decide upon the quantity.

You also need to know whether a percentage of the cost can be covered under your health insurance or not. For example, medicines made and produced by pharmaceutical companies will no doubt have FDA approval. However, marijuana in its raw form has no such approval. The FDA considers marijuana to have a high potential for abuse and will not therefore approve it on the basis that they feel it has no medical use.

Although the American Medical Association is pushing for a change in the classification of marijuana, the equivalent of half a dozen joints can cost the user between $25 and $60. Some dispensaries do give discounted marijuana for medical use to people of low income, though this is not uniform and cannot always be counted upon.

Thus, using marijuana for medical purposes can be expensive and users have been known to spend up to $1000 a month on it because no relief is available for them and no insurance companies are reimbursing the cost even though the marijuana has been approved for medical purposes.

This is another reason why you may find it an incentive to grow your own, though please do check the chapter which covers this, since there may be restrictions on the amount you are allowed to grow.

At the end of the day, all medicines cost money. If you do find a supplier at a reasonable price that gives you good quality marijuana that is grown organically, there's no price you can actually put on good health. It may be worthwhile from that perspective and patients may be able to make other economies in their lives that allow for this non insurable aspect of medical use of marijuana.

The types of products which may be covered under your health plan would be those medications which either imitate the effect of marijuana or those which contain the THC but in a recognized pill or liquid format sold by pharmaceutical companies.

Look into this aspect with your insurer and do discuss need with your local health provider, as there may be assistance available for those with great need of this kind of medical help.

CHAPTER SEVEN

HOW DOES MEDICAL MARIJUANA COMPARE TO OTHER PAIN MEDICATIONS?

You may be wondering why go through all the hassle of looking for marijuana when you can simply buy other pain medications that may be very easy to purchase at the pharmacy. Despite being able to access pain medications easily, it's important to be aware of the side effects and addictive nature of many of the pain medications on the market so that you can make an informed decision.

Common side effects to pain medications include:

- ❖ Abdominal pain
- ❖ Inflammation and destruction of kidneys
- ❖ Lethargy
- ❖ Hypothermia
- ❖ Heavy sweating
- ❖ Nausea and vomiting
- ❖ Mood changes
- ❖ Confusion and seizures
- ❖ Dizziness, hearing loss and vision disturbances
- ❖ Constipation
- ❖ Addiction

The symptoms highlighted above are not to scare you but to inform you on the potential side effects of pain medications. This is in no way to make you turn to using marijuana, since marijuana also has its own side effects. The goal is to enable you make an informed decision based on knowledge of pain medication and the adverse effects it can have.

On TV, you may have seen people steal pain medication following addiction to it. This is common with pain medication which is taken long term and doctors try to wean patients off it gradually so as to avoid the addiction setting in. One can understand why the addiction occurs. First there is the fear of the pain. The painkillers help to alleviate that fear but they do more than that. They make the pain go away. Thus, those on painkillers come to depend upon the pills to stop the pain and are often afraid to stop taking them, long after the pain has actually been dealt with because they fear the pain coming back. This psychological fear is very real and can lead to addiction.

Marijuana also has its own pitfalls. For instance, you may experience a sore throat as a result of ongoing use, or you may find difficulty breathing occasionally similar to that experienced with smoking cigarettes. Eating or vaporizing marijuana rather than smoking it can deal with this problem. Consumption of marijuana also causes short-term memory loss, although once the herb wears off, any memory problems are regained.

Marijuana can cause a hunger that is well known by those who consume marijuana and is commonly known as "the munchies" although this isn't disadvantageous because it can give people an appetite boost after illness that may actually increase the rapidity of recovery. In normal use, perhaps having healthy "munchies" as opposed to the chocolate flavored munchies preferred by regular smokers, this may also help patients to be aware of their food intake and change their lifestyle habits for healthier ones.

In doing a comparison between pharmaceutical drugs for pain and marijuana, those that are manufactured by pharmaceutical companies will have many side effects. If you read the notice that comes with many drugs, these are diverse, whereas the side effects from marijuana are less likely to mess up the digestion or to need other medications to counter the side effects.

It's kind of a vicious circle thing. When taking medicines for pain, one has to weigh up the potential of what damage they do to other parts of the body and what remedial action is needed to counter those effects. With marijuana, it's just a question of how the drug will be taken, and deciding upon how often it is needed. As marijuana may make you a little lethargic, you also need to choose times that do not disrupt your lifestyle.

Driving

When comparing pharmaceutical painkillers with marijuana, you have to take into account a lot of variances. Both can affect the ability to concentrate, the motor coordination and indeed the reaction times that are necessary for good driving practice.

If you read the details of painkillers prescribed, it's quite possible that this is warned against on packets of extra strong pain medications. Even those that are sold over the counter can affect the ability to drive depending upon the individual and their response to that medication.

In the case of those smoking marijuana, there are studies that indicate a rise in the potential of accidents while driving, but this also applies to alcohol and to prescription medications. The common sense indicator is that if you find your level of concentration is insufficient to drive, and then avoiding driving is the sensible option, whether this lack of concentration is caused by prescription medication, alcohol or by marijuana. Other drugs which spring to mind immediately are anti-depressants and medications given to people having psychiatric treatment.

The side effects of Marinol that is a synthetic THC are dizziness, drowsiness and light-headedness. These symptoms may diminish after being on the treatment for a while, though as stated earlier in the book, it's a great shame that natural marijuana was rejected in favor of Marinol in the treatment of cancer patients who suffered vomiting after their cancer medications, since marijuana did prove to be more effective.

The common sense approach is that either traditional treatments for pain or marijuana do have side effects, but you need to measure these and be aware of your own capabilities before putting yourself into situations that are potentially dangerous. If a drug states that it can potentially make you feel dizzy, then common sense would tell you not to drive. In the same way, if marijuana use makes you feel dizzy then the best course of action is to avoid driving until your composure is regained and you are able to drive without added risk.

Marijuana does not come with a notice that gives you the side effects and these differ with every individual that uses it. It's much like when you see a list on a pharmaceutical drug; you can see what kind of side effects to expect. In the case of marijuana, it's better to err on the side of caution until you are aware of the side effects is causes in your particular instance, as someone else's experience will not be your experience.

Start with a small amount and adjust this as and when you know what amount is useful to you, and what amount is likely to make you too tired to function correctly. If you overstepped the mark with prescription medications, it's exactly the same. You can overdo it. Cautious use will show you how much marijuana you actually need to make you feel better.

Once you know this, you are better able to know how much you need to purchase and how long that has to last you, bearing in mind your financial situation.

Traditional pain medications can be abused. If you take too many, you are likely to become very dependent upon having a regular supply. Even though these may be legal and may be refunded by your health insurance, they may not be doing your body the best service they can long term. Marijuana, on the other hand, tackles your stress levels without leaving you with that yearning for chemicals that you experience with traditional pain medication.

CHAPTER EIGHT

THC VS. CBD

Δ9-tetrahydrocannabinol (THC) is the most popular and most extensively studied in the science of cannabis. However, in the recent past, cannabidiol (CBD) is in the foreground due to its capacity to provide therapeutic relief for children suffering from epilepsy. CBD is usually preferred due to its inability to make you high, as explained in the previous chapter. Despite THC often being preferred for its induced feelings of euphoria, and CBD for its sedative properties, both compounds along with 66 other cannabinoids are considered useful for treating various conditions.

Cannabis contains elements that can briefly be described as the "Big Six": CBD, THC, THCV CBN, CBC and CBG.

Any cannabis plant contains these and many other cannabinoids in different proportions, forming the overall chemical profile of the plant. Chemically, the cannabis plant has many other compounds like proteins, fatty acid esters, sugars, amino acids, enzymes and flavonoids among others.

The Entourage

Generally, all these compounds are important in providing the relief you may be looking for. So how do these compounds provide therapeutic relief? The answer is found in a concept called "the effect of the entourage."

Initially described in 1998 by Israeli scientists, Shabbat Shimon, Ben-Rafael and Meshullam, the concept of the effect of the entourage simply means that the cannabinoids in the cannabis plant work together synergistically. Many studies have actually indicated that whole plant extracts are more effective as compared to using THC alone. Wilkinson and colleagues studies confirmed that the whole plant extracts are more effective than THC alone. The "entourage" or whole is therefore preferred for therapeutic medical use, rather than the THC on its own, which is the part of the cannabis plant which gives the feeling of being "high."

The effect of the entourage can also make cannabis extracts effective in the treatment of various bacterial infections. There are a number of studies showing antibacterial properties of cannabinoids. The World Health website tells of how cannabinoids destroyed the super bug MRSA. These cannabinoids are not psychotropic or do not contain any kind of mood altering ability, but that they can kill bacteria, thus stopping MRSA in its tracks from developing. The study of this aspect of cannabis really does need more research since the potential is enormous.

Finally, the effect of the entourage allows specific cannabinoids to modify or reduce the negative side effects of other cannabinoids. The most relevant example of this is the ability to modify the CBD, reducing the negative effects of THC.

Many patients have heard of (or experienced) the increased anxiety and paranoia that are sometimes associated with cannabis. Due to the effect of the entourage, the study shows that CBD can help minimize the anxiety associated with THC and lower paranoia.

As can be seen, THC, CBD, and other cannabinoids do not compete but rather work in tandem with the other extracts in order to provide therapeutic relief for a wide range of diseases. Nature always gives the best answer and this is no exception with the cannabis plant because the whole plant gives more therapeutic value than any extracted part of the plant.

CHAPTER NINE

WHAT CAN MARIJUANA TREAT?

Various illnesses can be treated with marijuana. Some speculate that marijuana can actually cure cancer and AIDS. Although these may be popular opinion, they have not yet been proven and people need to take medications of a more traditional nature until proof is obtained that marijuana does have any effect in cases as serious as cancer and AIDS. It is well known that marijuana is used to reduce vomiting after a patient is subjected to cancer treatment. There are also treatments that are synthetic which are offered to these patients, based on their closeness in characteristics to marijuana.

The list of the diseases for which one can take a prescription for the usage of marijuana is different in many states. However, Dr. Tod Mikuriya, a psychiatrist and an advocate for the legalization of marijuana, has compiled a list of the variety of illnesses that can be treated by medical marijuana, as proven by scientific research. This shows an interesting and diverse range of uses to which marijuana can be put to help patients to feel better or to reduce risks of illnesses. Some of them are:

Reduces growth in tumor formations
Research has shown that cannabis helps to delay reproduction and slows down the production of cancerous cells in the body. In other words, cannabis reduces the growth of tumors. It is also a natural anti-emetic, which makes it effective in the inhibition of nausea and vomiting caused by chemotherapy and radiotherapy.

This is backed to a certain degree by a study that was done by the National Cancer Institute, though the study was done on rats and showed a decrease in certain types of tumor after various doses of THC. While responses were good in the case of breast cancer, there were also notes that cancer cell development was certainly affected by the introduction of THC. However, this shouldn't be translated as being something definite since more studies are needed before the correlation can truly be established between the use of cannabis by normal users and the reduction of cancer cells. Since normal users would not simply be ingesting THC, but all of the elements of marijuana, then there would seem to be a different set of circumstances.

Relieves symptoms of chronic pain

Cannabis is one of the best natural painkillers available, if not the best natural painkiller available. It can help those suffering from acute and chronic pain function at an optimum level. The effects are often much more pronounced than those of other, more conventional painkillers. There may be several reasons for this. Since the THC enters into the nervous system, it may help to cut pain signals and give the patient a feeling of well being that makes the pain less taxing to endure.

It may also be that the anti-bacterial effects of marijuana help to reduce potential swelling or inflammation that causes the pain in the first place. When pain occurs, particularly on a chronic and ongoing basis, the patient is likely to become tense, thus making the pain worse. However, with the introduction of marijuana, the pain lessens because the tenseness can be avoided.

Alzheimer's

Cannabis reduces the occurrence of depression in patients suffering from Alzheimer's disease. Reducing depression allows the patient to maintain a higher level of brain activity. This can be an extremely powerful method for maintaining functionality for a longer period of time.

There has been further research into the effect of THC on the progress of Alzheimer's disease and this seemed to show that there was a slowing down of the process of the illness when THC was introduced. The anti-inflammatory action of marijuana seemed to have a bearing on this disease, since it is known to be caused by inflammation of the brain. The research further showed that early smoking of marijuana might actually prevent Alzheimer's from actually occurring.

Glaucoma

Certain species of this herb can potentially reduce the amount of pressure that may be exerted on the optic nerve from glaucoma. There are those that argue that this relief only lasts for the time that the marijuana is active and that this can be limited to two or three hours, although the use of the plant for glaucoma dates back to the very beginning of time. The connection is strong enough to show that marijuana could potentially be used for long term treatment of glaucoma.

Prevents Epilepsy Attacks

Nearly 2 million Americans suffer epilepsy attacks every year. Epilepsy is a condition in which certain brain cells become extremely agitated. When using marijuana to control epilepsy, it's important to do so under a doctor's care. Medical marijuana isn't a substitute for other epilepsy medication and one should never stop taking medication without their doctor's recommendation.

However, research shows that certain strains of marijuana have anti-convulsive properties and are being used successfully, especially in children. Talk to a medical professional about this before taking for granted that this is the case for any child or for any adult. These are merely findings that need more looking into in the case of having epilepsy. However, the Epilepsy Council supports the findings that medical marijuana treatment improves the lives of people with epilepsy and reduces the amount of attacks suffered.

Hyperactivity disorders

Many people who suffer from hyperactivity disorders find that medical cannabis restores their ability to concentrate and improves their ability to function efficiently. Though there are no clinical studies in humans to prove this, some initial studies performed on animals indicated a reduction in hyperactivity and impulsiveness from the use of cannabinoids.

This is a fairly common sense use as marijuana is known to help people to "chill" out, or to relax and thus it may slow down the hyperactivity by the very nature of its potential to help the patient slow down and relax.

Soothes patients suffering from Tourette's syndrome and obsessive-compulsive disorder

Several physiological disorders are also associated with the medical benefits of cannabis. Regular intake of prescribed cannabis can slow tics for those who suffer from Tourette syndrome. It can also slow the obsessive thinking and compulsive behavior in obsessive compulsive disorder (OCD). Some of the qualities of the cannabis plant help manage disturbing thoughts that cause fear, anxiety, or an excited state. However one should be aware that used in some cases, it can also cause paranoia. It's not so much a question of how much is taken, but in what circumstances and by who since different people will react to it in different ways. Much of the paranoia may be because of the illegality of the drug or the feeling of guilt, though one could say the same thing for pharmaceutical drugs given for depression and other mental illnesses.

Chronic pain and fibromylgia

In cases such this, marijuana is used to cut down the inflammation that causes the pain. As a proven anti-inflammatory agent, marijuana is preferable to pharmaceutical anti-inflammatory medications, since there are none of the side effects common to those drugs. For example, those taking anti-inflammatory drugs to ease pain may also have to take other drugs to counter the bad side effects. Side effects commonly caused by medical treatments for inflammation include problems with the digestive system. This can be avoided by use of cannabis, as opposed to the standard treatments.

There are many illnesses that can use marijuana to help patients in different ways. Those illnesses that involve a lot of pain can be helped considerably with the use of marijuana, as can any of the illnesses shown below which relate to inflammation of any sort, which is reduced with the use of marijuana. In the case of some of the serious ailments such as Hepatitis C and cancer, the help that is offered by marijuana is as an aid to stem to side effects of traditional medications, which are known to be hard for patients to deal with.

❖ Shingles

❖ Premenstrual Syndrome (PMS)

❖ Hepatitis

- ❖ Inflammatory Bowel Disease

- ❖ Endometriosis

- ❖ Diabetes

- ❖ Migraines / Headaches

- ❖ Arthritis

- ❖ Autoimmune diseases

- ❖ Neuropathic pain

- ❖ Cancer - including skin, prostate, brain, colon, lung, ovarian, leukemia, etc.

- ❖ Back pain

Different marijuana strains for treating various conditions

With so many marijuana strains available it is easy to confuse the strain and which one is the most appropriate strain for your ailment. For instance, the most suitable strain for chronic pain is Afghan and Big bud. When experiencing frequent headaches and migraines, the most suitable option is Super Lemon Haze or White gold. In case you are experiencing pain in your joints and nothing seems to work, you may use Purple Kush. White widow, Apollo 11, and Black Domina are the best when having muscle spasms. If chemotherapy is taking a toll on you, consider using Cinderella 99. Blueberry is the best when dealing with depression.

What should be borne in mind that all over the world, people have different names for the strains of marijuana and it may be necessary, if you are reading this from anywhere other than the United States that you check the name given against the strains available in your geographical area.

There is a very comprehensive guide to all of the different strains shown on this web page, which may be useful for those who are thinking of beginning to take marijuana in response to an illness being suffered.

CHAPTER TEN

MEDICAL MARIJUANA AND CANCER

One of the primary points that have been emphasized in the book is marijuana's use for cancer patients. Medical marijuana time and again has been researched with its role in cancer treatment. Many debates have been raise and legality issues discussed with regard to marijuana being used to help with effects of chemotherapy and such.

Marijuana has actually been an herbal remedy since a long time in history. They are classified as Schedule I controlled substances. This means that it is not FDA approved or legally prescribed. Although there are the two drugs made from its THC component have been approved by the FDA as a treatment.

It is legal in almost twenty-three states as well.

However the use of marijuana is still frowned upon in many places. In cancer treatment, its elements such as THC and CBD have been researched on and they have been deemed to be quite effective as well.

THC is known to be responsible for the 'high' that most users experience. It is the compound that helps relieve can help relieve pain and nausea, reduce inflammation, and can act as an antioxidant. While Cannabidiol (CBD) can help treat seizures, can reduce anxiety and paranoia, and can counteract the dizziness caused by THC.

Effects vary based on the way that it has been taken. For example if it's by mouth the process is slow and effects produced are different from when it's taken through vaporization. In vaporization the process is quick and effects fade faster than when it is taken through the mouth.

When it comes to cancer treatment, a number of studies regarding smoked marijuana found that it could be helpful in treating nausea and vomiting from cancer chemotherapy. A few studies have also shown that inhaled marijuana can be very helpful in treatment of neuropathic pain (pain caused by damaged nerves). Other studies have shown that people who took marijuana extracts in clinical trials showed less dependency on pain medicine. More recently, scientists reported that THC and other cannabinoids such helped slow growth and even cause death in certain types of cancer cells. Some animal studies also suggest certain cannabinoids may restrict growth and reduce spread of some forms of cancer.

Even lung cancer patients can use medical marijuana; studies show that smoking marijuana is not a cause for cancer growth. Research has also shown that marijuana slows the effects of cervical cancer and lung cancer. Cannabidiol, one of the five cannabinoids found in medical marijuana, also restricts tumor growth in leukemia and breast cancer. Patients undergoing cancer treatment often use medical marijuana to reduce vomiting and nausea, and it has presented itself as very effective in that purpose.

In a review presented by the University of Arkansas on the development of breast cancer, it was revealed that cannabinoids could be a treat vomiting and nausea in cancer patients after surgery.

In addition, medicinal marijuana is also helpful with cancer related weight loss. It can serve as an appetite stimulant to improve treatment induced anorexia.

Research is also ongoing to discover further effects of marijuana in cancer patients.

Drugs

Dronabinol or Marinol is a capsule containing tetrahydrocannabinol (THC) and is approved by the US Food and Drug Administration (FDA). It can be administered to treat nausea and vomiting caused by cancer chemotherapy; it also works well for weight loss and as a cure for poor appetite in patients with AIDS.

Nabilone is a synthetic cannabinoid that acts much like THC. It can be taken by mouth to treat vomiting caused by cancer chemotherapy. It has proved to be efficient when other drugs have failed to treat patients.

In UK, there is Sativex. But it is only used for treatment in spasms and pain in patients of Multiple Sclerosis (MS).

Nabiximols is a cannabinoid drug still under study in the US. It's a mouth spray made up of a plant extract with THC and CBD put together in a ratio of almost one to one as a mixture. It's available in

Canada and parts of Europe to treat pain linked to cancer, as well as muscle spasms and pain from multiple sclerosis. It's not approved in the US as of 2015, but it's being tested in clinical trials.

All these drugs have known to be helpful in cancer treatment. But do not forget that they also come with side effects. So it is necessary that a patient consult their oncologist when trying out marijuana as a treatment.

Side effects can be dizziness, mood disorders, heart and blood related problems. It also depends upon the age. As to what age bracket a person belongs to. Elderly people might exhibit different side effects than younger people.

The American Cancer Society (AMA) has also presented their stance as far as marijuana's use is concerned. It supports the need for more scientific research on cannabinoids for cancer patients. It recognizes the need for better and more effective therapies that can provide relief and help with the physically and mentally damaging side effects of cancer and its treatment.

The society is against the classification of marijuana as a Schedule I controlled substance and argues that it imposes numerous conditions on researchers. It restricts and prevents scientific study of chemicals and compounds in marijuana.

Medical decisions about pain and symptom management should be made between the patient and his or her doctor. The choice should be made by scrutinizing evidence of benefit and harm to the patient. The patient's preferences and values should be considered along with any laws and regulations that may apply.

Even the National Institute of Drug Abuse has given their revised report of marijuana's medical abilities. Their report has shown that in animals, it has restricted and stunted the growth of cancer cells. Other studies were conducted on mice and the results were that marijuana was increasingly helpful with the treatment of serious tumors. Apart from that, when it was conducted along with radiation, it even propelled the killing of cancer cells.

Cannabis, it has been discovered can help with many types of cancer such as lung cancer, leukemia, brain cancer, cervical cancer, breast cancer and more.

According to a study, the component cannabinol possesses a unique healing compound that has the capability to hinder the progress of the gene that is responsible for the spread of cancer. At the same time, it does not even have the psychological effects that area result of marijuana smoking. It can prevent cancer in addition to reducing diabetes and heart attacks by fifty-eight and sixty-six percent respectively.

This study was made by a Spanish group of medical experts and is not validated by any American group.

The Spanish medical team conducted the tests on glioblastoma multiform cancer that is one of the most difficult cancers to treat. It often does not respond to conventional cancer treatment such as surgery, chemotherapy and radiotherapy. They wanted to see whether cutting off blood supply through the use of medical marijuana could stop its growth.

The results came to show that the genes that are associated with blood vessel growth in a tumor had their activity greatly reduced. The genes produced which had its production cut off by certain components in Cannabinol.

Aside from treating one of the most difficult cancers, it is shown to be highly effective in treating non-melanoma cancer. Non-melanoma cancer is usually considered to be one of the most common malignancies found among people. Given the growth stunting effects of cannabinol on cancer cells glioblastoma, scientists started studying the potential capabilities of these elements in skin cancer tumor therapy.

The results were surprisingly positive. Cannabinol stimulated receptors that could cause skin cancer cell death. At the same time, it was found to stop the progression of the cancer causing epidermal cells. The study also shows that marijuana can decrease activity in skin tumor components, especially in one compound that plays a vital role in causing the growth of blood vessels that stimulate skin tumor growth.

Other than these benefits, medical marijuana also helps cancer patients who have trouble in getting sleep. It also helps stimulates a person's fading sense of smell and taste post chemotherapy. Marijuana might be responsible for causing a couple of disorders and anxiety. But few can say that it causes lack of sleep or insomnia.

Whether they are responding to treatment or not, or dealing with the aftermath of the diagnosis, insomnia is not a matter fun for anyone. The cannabinol found in medical marijuana has often been shown to help with relaxation. A patient who is dealing with being diagnosed with cancer is obviously having trouble sleeping, and it assists them in falling asleep easier and faster. Sleep is a vital part of any kind of a recovery process. If the human body is unable to recuperate properly, it will often experience difficulties in the process of curing itself.

At the same time, medical marijuana is helpful in dealing with dizziness as well. Many patients who undergo cancer treatment often find that they get dizzy and lose focus. Medical marijuana has been found to actually help patients who suffer from these symptoms, which in turn also reduces vomiting caused by them

As a chain reaction, it further helps the individual keep their food down and even gain weight, and that is an important factor in recovery.

CHAPTER ELEVEN

MEDICAL MARIJUANA AND MENTAL HEALTH

Marijuana has usually been associated adversely as being the cause of mental problems. It is considered as a reason for deteriorating mental health in frequent users and campaigners against its use cite this as a major reason for why it should not be legalized.

There are two sides to this. While yes, it can be the cause of disorders, it can also provide help with some. Due to restricted research due to state laws and prohibitions of use, scientists have been unable to study on its full potential as a cure to mental disorders.

Within the limited studies, results have been deduced that show that marijuana can be of help with PTSD (Post-Traumatic Syndrome Disorder), OCD (Obsessive Compulsive Disorder) and Depression.

A study on rats conducted by the University of Buffalo's Research Institute on Addictions has pointed to the possibility that certain components in marijuana may help with the treatment of stress related depression.

A study that came in The Journal of Neuroscience, focused on endocannabinoids. These are chemicals in the brain quite similar to the chemicals found in marijuana that are known as cannabinoids. These are involved in memory, mood, pain sensations and appetite. They're also involved with the psychological effects that cannabis has on us. It also influences brain functions such as cognition, behavior, and emotions.

The researchers found that in animal models, chronic stress led less production of endocannabinoids, which in turn became a cause of depressive symptoms.

A senior researcher at the institute stated that chronic stress was one of the major causes of depression. And marijuana can be used to replenish the production of endocannabinoid due the similarity between the compounds.

The compounds derived from cannabis to restore normal function could potentially help in stabilizing moodiness and release depression. The study cannot be validated as it is yet to be tested on humans.

However there have been other studies that find that compounds in cannabis such as THC have also been known to eliminate depression.

There has been a strong debate as to whether marijuana can really help improve mental health or not.

While some medical experts agree that it is why there are fewer disorders among teenagers and suicide rate is decreasing, there are others who argue that it actually worsens problems and lead to a poor mental stability.

CHAPTER TWELVE

MEDICAL MARIJUANA AND EPILEPSY

As discussed in the book a few times, one of marijuana's recently discovered properties is the ability to help control epileptic seizures.

Researchers say that it has actually been known for some time now that marijuana can help with epilepsy and its symptoms. Research dating from the 1980's has been found and it contains evidence that medical cannabis can help ease the seizures in epileptic patients.

Recently, the issue came to light due to the documentary 'Weed' that aired in 2013. Here filmmaker Sanjay Gupta recorded the case of a five year old girl Charlotte Figi, who suffered from Dravet's Syndrome. This Colorado native suffered from violent, frequent seizures. However after being administered with medical marijuana, the seizures registered a dramatic drop and were almost stopped. She even recovered from developmental delays being caused by the disease. There was a major outcry that followed this discovery.

After watching the documentary "Weed," many parents of children with epilepsy throughout the United States became aware of the treatment that marijuana could provide. They began to rally for the easy access to medical marijuana. And when faced with resistance from their elected representatives to allow access to medical marijuana by passing laws, many of the desperate families moved. They went to Colorado and other states, where medical marijuana is readily available.

These people were termed as 'medical marijuana refugees'. They joined the families of epileptic children along with many other patients who suffering from other serious illnesses in recognizing the demand for this medicine. They ask for it to be made easily accessible to those who need it.

Life threatening Epilepsy

There are many known forms of epilepsy that can affect children at a very early age, even when they are babies and infants. These include Doose syndrome, Lennox Gastaut syndrome, Dravet's syndrome and development of early epilepsy. They all result in frequent convulsions, which ultimately cause cognitive and behavioral impairment, along with movement delays.

There are some children who experience up to a hundred seizures per day, some lasting as long as half an hour. This makes regular function for them highly impossible. The mortality rate is high, almost up to fifteen and twenty percent by a young age only. Commonly most deaths are known to occur during sleep due to a phenomenon that is called sudden unexplained death in epilepsy (sudep).

It was even reported that in an unfortunate event, one young child in New Jersey recently died. She and her family were waiting for her application for medical marijuana, which is legal in that state, to be approved.

Cannabidiol (CBD)

Recently, there have been a number of open labeled (patients know about the treatment being given) studies in the U.S. of Epidiolex (a drug derived from cannabidiol or CBD), which is produced by a pharmaceutical company (GW Pharmaceuticals). Epidiolex is a purified, oil-based extract of CBD that is produced and given in known and consistent amounts in each dose. The U.S. Food and Drug Administration (FDA) even gave some epilepsy centers permission to administer this drug as a 'compassionate use' for a limited number of people at each center.

Such studies are ongoing to find positive results for difficult epilepsies such as Lennox-Gastaut syndrome (in children and adults) and Dravet syndrome in children.

Results from over two hundred people who received Epidiolex in an open label study that was without a placebo control were presented at the American Academy of Neurology on April 22nd, 2015 in Washington DC. Data from a hundred and thirty-seven people who completed twelve weeks or more on the drug was analyzed. It was used to look at how helpful or effective the drug had been. People who received the Epidiolex fell in the bracket from age to twenty-six years old with an average age of eleven.

All had epilepsy that was not responding to any other treatment currently available. Approximately twenty-five to eighteen percent had Dravet Syndrome (DS) and twenty-two to sixteen percent were suffering from Lennox-Gastaut Syndrome (LGS).

The news that it had been effective for some children with hard core epilepsy who have been given a marijuana strain rich in cannabidiol (CBD) spread fast in this day and age of technology. And it led to parents of children with epilepsy desperately trying to obtain more information about medical marijuana and provide their children with a chance to try the treatment.

Despite fears that marijuana extracts rich in CBD can increase the risk of psychological disorders and long term problems, people are tending to focus on the positives. Let's face it; every kind of medicine comes with its due side effects.

The positive impact on some people with epilepsy that has been recorded as a result of taking CBD and marijuana extracts have given so many families searching for proper treatment, hope.

The results that were observed in the study of epilepsy were:

- ❖ Seizures registered a decrease by an average of fifty-four percent in a hundred and thirty-seven people who completed twelve weeks on Epidiolex.

- ❖ Patients who had DS (Dravet's syndrome) responded even more positively with a sixty-three percent decrease in seizures over three months.

- ❖ This improvement in seizures lasted through twenty-four weeks on the Epidiolex, more often for people with DS than without DS.

- ❖ In twenty-seven patients with the chronic seizures, there was a decrease of 66.7% in them on average.

- ❖ The responder rate (the number of people whose seizures decreased by at least 50%) was also observed as being slightly better in patients with DS (about 55% at three months) as compared to patients without DS (50%).

- ❖ There were people who were also taking the medicine Clobazam (Onfi) and they seemed to respond more favorably to the Epidiolex. There was a greater improvement in convulsive seizures within those patients than in patients who were not taking Clobazam. Experts suggested that an interaction between Clobazam and Epidiolex might have played a part in the differences seen.

In the same study, the initiators and administrators also noted the side effects that came with it:

- ❖ Diarrhea
- ❖ Sleepiness
- ❖ Fatigue
- ❖ Less appetite

All those side effects were noticed in a percentage of people from seventeen to twenty-one percent.

Around ten people (5%) stopped treatment with Epidiolex due to side effects, though three of these people came back and restarted it. Most side effects were described as mild or moderate and went away.

Serious side effects were presented in fifty-two people and twenty-two of those were possibly because of their relation to the drug. The most common serious side effect that was possibly present is known as status epilepticus. This is when a person has long or repeated seizures.

Two people even died while taking Epidiolex, although the deaths were not thought to be related to the drug.

A few children also had to change their seizure medication in order to lessen sleepiness and the sedative effect. Interactions between Epidiolex and certain seizure medications were found to be the cause of changes in blood levels of seizure medications. It was occurring in small numbers of people and was noted in an earlier report of this study.

It is difficult to properly and extensively assess the side effects of Epidiolex and other epilepsy medicines. Safety concerns cannot become evident until larger studies using a control group are done. Other side effects could occur that are simply not known yet to practicing physicians. This and its potential efficacy as an epilepsy cure are two of the most important reasons as to why rigorous clinical trials are needed.

Many people who have severe epilepsy are known to try a number of mind numbing medications, surgeries, implanted, diets and alternative therapies. But they get very little relief in their symptoms. While yes, there may be some harmful side effects from these marijuana extracts, but compared against the dangers and challenges that a child or even an adult with seizures faces every day, there are outweighed. There may seem no other option left.

Like every other argument, there are two sides to this as well. The ones against it can say that different reactions can result within different people. Some may boast of positive results while some may show negative ones due marijuana containing dangerous components.

It could be said that the THC component can actually trigger some seizures in addition to other adverse psychoactive effects including depression and neurosis that can also occur with the use of marijuana. Also, the withdrawal effects of marijuana on seizure activity have not been well studied. A person could be at a higher risk for seizures as marijuana is metabolized or if someone stops using marijuana all together.

Apart from that, nobody really knows how marijuana can affect the anti-epileptic medication already circulating within blood levels. Many lethal and harmful ingested substances can alter levels of antiepileptic medications sometimes leading to increases seizures or toxic side effects.

Use of marijuana can negatively affect memory (which is also a well-known side effect of many antiepileptic drugs) that in turn can lead to an upset in dosage of medicine or even altogether missing it. This might result in an increased risk of seizures.

Finally, there is the potential for pulmonary (lung) complications from the inhalation of marijuana if a person is using smoked form of it.

The people arguing in favor of it could counter it by supporting marijuana and listing its benefits in treating the disease. It is obvious that not everybody needs to be treated with it. Only in cases when the anti-epileptic drugs prescribed for these children do not work. Sometimes these drugs can even worsen these seizures. Many of the AEDs carry really harsh side effects, from moderate to even life threatening. Yes, maybe even worse that marijuana's.

Some of the milder side effects are insomnia, eye problems, hyperactivity and weight gain. Others include fainting and palpitations.

The major side effects that can lead to serious life threatening situations include peeling of large areas of the skin and blistering, both of these can result in hospitalization.

Parents of epileptic children have stated that they usually try many different medications but see no significant improvement. And many also become wary of the side effects that sometimes can be as destructive as the seizing.

In states where medical marijuana is legal, there were surveys conducted and it was reported that on an average, epileptic children and patients had tried up to twelve various medications before resorting to medical cannabis.

Medical marijuana is also known for possessing properties that prevent convulsion. Most of the anticonvulsant properties come from the chemical in the plant called CBD (Cannabidiol). While the need for more detailed research is there, some scientific evidence has been discovered that suggests that cannabis and its extracts can reduce seizures and may also have less damaging side effects.

It is easy to administer amongst children with seizure disorders. In Colorado it was shown that the children took medical marijuana in the form of an oil solution containing high CBD cannabis extract. It can be put under the tongue or in a feeding tube as well. This particular extract has a high content of CBD is called as the 'Charlotte's Web'. It carries very low levels of THC, and parents report that their children do not experience any mentally altering effects. They also report no negative side effects.

In fact there are several positive effects as well, aside from reducing seizures. Parents report that their children are sleeping better sleep, have mood stability and overall alertness.

Doctors also support it. There were three neurologists at the University of Utah's Division of Pediatric Neurology. The division Chief Dr. Francis Fallout, who specializes in Dravet syndrome, along with those neurologists expressed support for it. The Chief even recently wrote to the Utah Controlled Substances Advisory Committee regarding the matter.

He wrote that he would like to express his strong desire that the drug of epilepsy become available to all children in Utah. He believed that the substance was not 'psychoactive or hallucinogenic' and that it contains less THC do other drugs. He argued that there was no potential of abuse with this.

They join a growing group of medical practitioners who are urging legal access of marijuana. There is the Epilepsy Foundation and experts on their Board, like Dr. Orrin Devinksy, who advocate for legalization. Devinsky recently wrote that as a doctor, he would definitely prescribe marijuana for many patients if it were legal in the state.

Despite of its negativities it shows results and has helped many desperate families. It's a promising treatment for some people. If given the scope of further research, scientists would no doubt desire to run further tests on pure CBD, along with different combinations of THC and CBD mixed together in alternating low and high quantities.

However, this research takes time and that is one thing that many of these children with unrelenting seizures cannot afford to lose. This will lead to parents and families willing to go to any length in order to help their children. They will do everything in their power to try all possible treatments. This is because everybody knows the long term effects of uncontrolled seizures. These include worsening condition, mental disabilities, and sometimes even death.

Studies might take years to produce results and that is fine. But in the meantime compassionate use of marijuana should be granted to patients suffering from severe epilepsy.

CHAPTER THIRTEEN

HOW TO USE MEDICAL MARIJUANA

Smoking Marijuana

An effective and quick way to introduce cannabinoids into the bloodstream is through inhaling smoke from a pipe, bong or joint. Once you inhale the smoke, psychoactive effects or rather being "high" will be noticeable within three minutes. The amount of time that it takes for this to happen varies from person to person, but this state can last for up to several hours based on the strain.

Smoking is the most effective way to introduce cannabis into the body, but according to research that was undertaken by the University of Colorado Cancer Center, the smoke may be carcinogenic. The research indicated that THC on its own does not have any cancer causing compounds; however, the smoke from burning cannabis is carcinogenic. What this means is that the cannabis plant by itself is not carcinogenic. Although there is not enough evidence for a link between cannabis smoke and lung cancer, exposure to smoke of any kind for a long time can cause a decline in pulmonary functions.

Increasing the potency of the marijuana is a great way to reduce the amount of smoke inhaled. For instance, some derived concentrates like hash enable users to smoke less of the plant materials owing to the high levels of cannabinoids.

People who smoke marijuana tend to mix the marijuana with tobacco and this can increase the risk of cancer, as tobacco is well known for having links with cancer. There is also increased risk of heart problems due to the effect of tobacco on the arteries.

Vaporizing Cannabis

Are you concerned about using cannabis because of the smoke? You can consider vaporizing cannabis instead. Through vaporization, cannabinoids are released in a gas state from the use of heat without combustion. Vaporization does not produce the byproducts of combustion, like carbon monoxide and tar, which occur with smoking. Actually, the vapor that is released is much cooler than smoke, which makes it less damaging to your throat and lungs. If you need to know more about this method, then it's worthwhile finding out about vaporizing machines available in your area. These are one way that the drug can be used very effectively with the added bonus that you are not damaging your lungs to the same extent. If you are put off using medical marijuana because of the effects of smoke, this may be a way that you will find satisfactory.

Cannabis Edibles

Quite a number of those who use medical marijuana are turning to cannabis infused into foods. Simply cook foods and use marijuana as one of the ingredients. Marijuana infused foods includes cakes, cookies, candies and brownies. Butter is usually infused with cannabis, and then added to the normal recipe. The amount that you use will vary upon your own particular tastes or experience of use and experimentation will tell you the best quantities to use. medicalmarijuana.ca has some recipes that may help you to get started as these are very easy to follow.

The edibles are introduced into the body through the gastrointestinal tract and are actually processed by the liver. The liver breaks THC down into a component having sedative properties, making it suitable for patients with insomnia or those who have trouble relaxing.

The effects of cannabis after consumption of cannabis edibles are usually felt within an hour, lasting for six to ten hours. While cannabis edibles may seem preferable to smoking cannabis, the unpredictable strength can pose a problem. There are too many variables for this to be something that is predictable.

The strength of the edible is normally determined by the quantity and quality of marijuana. Furthermore, the effects of cannabis usually take longer to manifest after the consumption of an edible. Many factors determine how quickly the effects will occur: empty stomach, digestion rate, liver metabolism, etc. and you need to take into account that overcooking the edibles may also affect the efficiency of the marijuana.

Many patients eat more because the effects haven't occurred as quickly as they expected, leading to a higher intake than intended. It is advised to take one edible at a time and wait for around 1 hour or more for the effects before having a second dose. Otherwise, you could find that you get too lethargic and are unable to keep a record of correct quantities and effects. If you randomly eat cookies, for example, you are unable to establish how much marijuana is needed to actually achieve the goal intended.

Just imagine having pain, consuming a cookie with some marijuana in it, and getting total pain relief. That would be something to really be happy about and therefore, if you want to achieve the best results for your body, be very consistent with your measurements, so that you can reproduce what helped you the first time.

While the effects of the marijuana may take a while to be manifested, it is likely to be less tedious compared to smoking. This can beneficial, especially if you are in a public place and smoking is out of the question. In any case, you will not expose yourself to all the harmful side effects associated with smoking marijuana but you will need to be careful about your recipe ingredients in order to get consistent results.

Consumption of marijuana edibles may not be suitable if you are suffering from a lack of appetite or are experiencing severe nausea and vomiting since you may end up vomiting before the marijuana can take effect. Thus, use of cookies in the case of cancer relief from vomiting is not advised.

You should always keep the edibles stored in a safe place, away from children and pets. You should also ensure that you know your own reactions before trying them when you are not at home.

Cannabis tinctures

Tinctures simply refer to an alcohol-based solution of dissolved cannabinoids. Cannabis tinctures are consumed as drops. Drops of liquid are placed under the tongue and are usually absorbed directly into the bloodstream and are quickly taken to the brain. This is quite similar to smoking and vaporization due to the speed in which the cannabis takes effect. Cannabis tinctures may also be used in food, although the liver will process them and it may take up to an hour or more to obtain relief. If you do use tinctures in food, then you need to be aware that the variables shown above for edibles will apply.

It is important that you seek advice from your marijuana provider or experiment until you find what works for you. Remember that experimentation will cost you money, so err on the low side rather than trying too much marijuana at one time.

Topicals

Did you know you could use marijuana topically? Using cannabis on the skin does not have psychoactive reactions since the cannabis does not reach the brain. Marijuana topicals are available in sprays, lotions, ointments balms and salves. Using marijuana topically can assist in proving effective for relief from the pain of arthritis, minor burns, chapped skin, muscle soreness, joint pain and swelling, tendinitis and many other ailments. Topical marijuana not only has anti-inflammatory properties, it may also act as an antibacterial agent, assisting in the healing of wounds. Thus carrying the balm with you will mean that you can use it in preference to more chemically based pharmaceutical products. Some people prefer this as a natural remedy for areas that benefit from topical application.

Hash

Collecting resins make hash from the female cannabis plant's flowers. The resin collected is then compressed into small blocks referred to as "ear wax", which you may eat, adds to tea or edibles, or even smoke. Hash normally has a high THC content, which encourages some to use it in order to reduce the need for higher cannabis use.

The only problem with this is that you do need to know that your supply is from a reliable source, since hash can be mixed with other things to make it look like you are buying more than you actually are. Another thing that you may find is that the goodness has been taken out of the hash before being sold to you and it's therefore vital to have confidence in your supplier. Organically grown suppliers are the best and local rather than imported hash with a known origin is better than taking chances with buying from dubious sources.

Cannabis tea

Are you aware that you can take cannabis tea? The process of making cannabis tea is similar to how any other tea is made; boil water and pour the leaves into a pot, allow it to steep for around an hour. Since THC is slightly soluble in hot water, you may need to add oil, butter or alcohol. This can be useful for people having difficulty swallowing food, decreased appetite, nausea, etc. Thus, this makes it a good treatment for those who are suffering from the after effects of cancer treatment, as well as those with digestive problems.

Cannabis Resin

This is made from the oils taken from the heads of the plants, which is shaped into a "soap" form or 9 bar (representing 9 ounces). Different countries have different names for it. The cannabis resin in this form is popular in Europe because it makes for easier transportation in block format. This cannabis is scraped from the piece bought into a pipe or into a hand rolled joint, though is commonly mixed with tobacco during this process in Europe. The color of the cannabis resin tends to give away its origin. That which comes from Pakistan has the nickname of "gold seal" because of the stamp that is used to show its authenticity. Its color is darker than other varieties. The lightest in color is Lebanese Gold although one should be aware that the strength gained from resins depends upon the voyage that the resin has taken, the age, the purity, the ambient temperature for the crop and transportation. There are so many variables that perhaps for medical use, this is not the best format. The other thing is that dealers can mix the resin with other content meaning that what the user ends up with is not pure. This is a general risk in the case of ever buying drugs that have an unknown origin as explained above.

CHAPTER FOURTEEN

SIDE EFFECTS OF MARIJUANA

You may be surprised to learn that Marijuana seems to be the safest psychoactive agent known to man because there is no established lethal dose for humans. Additionally, there are no known cases of disease or death as a direct result of its use. However, the association of marijuana use with use of more lethal illegal drugs has always been used as an excuse as to why marijuana should be legalized. In states where it has, it has also been recognized that if people can get their medical marijuana without coming into contact with dealers of more dangerous drugs, then this makes perfect sense. Other countries have looked into this as well, and the amount that they could make on taxes on marijuana may be the final deciding point in those countries currently considering it. This has been brought up in the side effects section because drugs in general have been given a bad reputation. Singled out and used on its own, marijuana's side effects are neither life threatening nor anything for a user to really be concerned about. It's important that new users know what the side effects may be, so that when they see these happening, they do not panic them.

One of the many side effects of marijuana, especially smoking marijuana, is an increased risk of respiratory disease due to the deposit of burnt plant materials into the lungs. This is increased when mixing marijuana with tobacco that is a known trigger for cancer. As well as damage to the lungs, it should be borne in mind that taking in marijuana in a smoked format may also cause throat irritation over a long period of time.

When inexperienced users try marijuana for the first time, they can experience anxiety. Rarely, this can escalate into a panic attack, accompanied by psychosomatic phenomena such as palpitations, choking, nausea, vomiting and collapse. In some cases, the use of marijuana may also lead to a state of paranoia manifested by delusions of persecution. There is evidence that this phenomenon is the result of the fear of punishment, fear of the drug, history of panic attacks, etc. although, as stated, this effect is rare. The illegality of the marijuana in some countries does cause paranoia to be more common, though more due to the fear of being caught than from the actual use of marijuana. Since marijuana heightens the senses, then it follows that those senses of worry would also be heightened. If you are concerned about panic attacks, then perhaps smoking with someone who knows how to use marijuana for medical purposes would be a good idea. This will help you learn how to use it, how to "go with the flow" and not to concentrate on the strange way that it feels which may in turn lead to paranoia or panic.

If you are going to use medical marijuana, treat it like any other medical drug. Talk to your doctor first, as he will have a history of your medical conditions and the medications that you are taking. He will also know whether you may be more prone to panic than other patients are. Discussing it will also give you the sense of knowing that what you have chosen as treatment is not counterproductive to any health condition you already have.

Consumption of marijuana can cause arrhythmia and an increase or decrease in blood pressure in patients with cardiovascular disease. It's always a good idea to keep your blood pressure measured. It's even worthwhile investing in a cuff that measures this so that you can adjust your pattern of lifestyle to help lower or increases your blood pressure naturally. Your actions do have a great deal of influence over how high or low your blood pressure is and this should be discussed with your general practitioner before taking medical marijuana, since he may know whether your medications are suited for use with marijuana.

Men may experience a temporary decrease in the levels of sex hormones and sperm count with consumption of marijuana, though this evidence is not conclusive. It is popular and while not proven to be a myth, may indicate that the best time to smoke medical marijuana is not when you are trying to grow your family. If you have any doubts, again it is advisable to talk with your doctor. Tests can be done to establish your sperm count, and if you find your sex drive is affected, you can adjust your medical marijuana intake so that you have days that are free of its use. As stated previously, this may not be an actual side effect, though until science provides full information, the precautions you use in your intake of medical marijuana help you to live a normal full life.

Other side effects of consumption of marijuana include lowered reaction time, increased heartbeat, short-term suppression of the immune system, reduced resistance to some common diseases like colds, inability to understand things clearly, mood swings, drowsiness, and sometimes reduced ability to retain information.

If you bear in mind the significance of the last paragraph, you will see that it is not sensible to drive or to operate machinery while under the influence of marijuana because lower reaction times can spell potential danger to both you and others. Thus, respecting this will help you to keep your use of marijuana for medical purposes safe and controlled.

CHAPTER FIFTEEN

MEDICAL MARIJUANA-
THE DEBATE

Marijuana or Cannabis as it is referred to, comes from the Cannabis plant as described earlier. In essence, it is a drug that can be used for health purposes as well as others. In medicine, it can be used primarily for improving appetite, help patients going through chemotherapy, for HIV patients and its most popular purpose, easing pain.

It is not yet that mainstream, as its legitimacy is a cause of debate in many countries. It has not been approved of as a legal drug for medical purposes by the FDA (Food and Drug Administration) and doctors are hesitant to prescribe it. Up till yet scientific study has only led to the approval of two medications found in pill form that contain cannabinoid chemicals.

There is ongoing research that might lead to further progress being made.

The cannabinoid chemicals that are found in marijuana are chemicals related to the THC. The THC is one of its main mind-effecting components. Other than that, a hundred other types of cannabinoids are found in medical marijuana. Scientists and researchers have tried to manufacture them in labs as well.

Many of these cannabinoids are powerful and can even have adverse effects on health. Interestingly enough the body also produces its own cannabinoid chemicals. These chemicals are responsible for regulating the five senses, pleasure, memory, awareness, and appetite and body movement.

Currently the two main interests of scientists in cannabinoid are THC and CBD. The THC reduces nausea and vomiting as mentioned previously well. The medicines are mainly approved for that purpose. While CBD is helpful with mental illnesses, pain and its most recently discovered purpose, controlling epileptic seizures.

Scientists and studies showed that purified extracts from the THC and CBD, when used with radiation could increase the cancer killing effects from the process.

Like in every debate there are two sides to this one as well. One lists the pros and the other counters it. Ultimately it is a matter of one's own judgment but these points can surely help a person come to decision as far as the medical use of marijuana is concerned.

PROS AND CONS

Physicians

Physicians have argued that there is clear evidence of its medical usefulness as far as pain relief and vomiting goes. It can be said that it is a safe drug and less toxic than others when it comes to the treatment of chronic illness such as MS (multiple sclerosis) or cancer.

While other experts have countered this by saying that there is no concrete data available that can show how effective it is. And the fact remain that it is a drug used for recreational purposes and can lead to harmful effects.

Medical Organizations

Another point made in favor of the medical marijuana has been raised by the ACP (American College of Physicians). Their report calls for a review for marijuana's classification and argues that it should be given a more appropriate status based on its medical efficacy.

In the report ACP has called for protection of physicians from prosecution and loss of licensing in case of prescribing medical marijuana. They have also cited protection of patients as long as state law permits them.

On the other hand, the NEI (National Eye Institute) came up with the premise that their studies conducted since 1978 had not shown any solid evidence of marijuana helping with glaucoma. And hence it is not that useful. In fact, its dangerous side effects were cited by them, like increased heart rate and decreased blood pressure.

U.S Government

An administrative DEA judge gave his approval to medical marijuana and supported his judgment by presenting evidence of its medical healing properties. He said that it helped a lot of very seriously ill people and was safely administered. Hence, the DEA should not stand between patients in need of this and should acknowledge its benefits in light of all the evidence.

While on the counter side, the director of the drug control policy office rejected any good side to marijuana. Marijuana was responsible for damage to integral organs in human body such as heart and lungs. It caused memory loss and impaired judgment. It was known to contain cancer causing elements and responsible for accidents and car crashes.

Health Risks of Smoked Marijuana

A Professor from Harvard University has argued that risks of smoking marijuana as a means of taking it to health are significantly less. Marijuana is being smoked over a number of countries world over and for quite some time. And as yet there have been no cases of lung cancer or any such life threatening disease that was inflicted mainly because of marijuana smoking.

He believes that a day of breathing polluted air of a metropolitan city can be more dangerous than smoking a portion of a join of marijuana.

Where else, a report from The British Lung Foundation finds the notion that marijuana smoke is harmless difficult to believe. The report says that smoking three to four cannabis cigarettes can have the same effect as smoking twenty or more tobacco cigarettes a day. It can severely damage bronchial mucosa and cause chronic or acute bronchitis.

It can become a cause of serious weakening of the immune system. Lung infections are caused by cell damage in the bronchial passage line and immune system ineffectiveness in the air sacs. The main reason for that could be cannabis smoking.

AIDS treatment with Marijuana

There are two sides to this as well. One report given by a doctor argues that patients receiving treatment through marijuana pills or smoking cannabis have shown improvement as compared to patients seeking other treatments. Patients receiving cannabinoid have registered a higher improvement in their immune system than patients who are receiving placebo.

They also gained more weight on average than the patients on placebo.

For the counter argument the report cited says that the most worrying concerns regarding marijuana smoking in HIV/AIDS patients are the possible effects of marijuana on immune system. Patients exhibiting fungal infections and bacterial pneumonia can lead to conclusions being derived that marijuana smoking can harm the immune system or exposes patients to other diseases.

It just basically means that patients who have deficiency in their immune system are likely to show vulnerability and harm that comes from marijuana smoking.

<u>For Terminally Ill</u>

For patients with terminal diseases, marijuana basically serves a therapeutic purpose. While one report is of the opinion that doctors and physicians should be able to easily prescribe this for such patients, the other one is against it.

The report for it suggests that marijuana actually helps these patients by easing pain and physicians should be compassionate and prescribe it for them. Its benefits have obviously outweighed the risks.

But the other one rejects the idea and says that it actually leeches away comfort in a patient's last days of life instead of providing them with it. Physicians should resort to other medicines to give relief and painlessness instead of marijuana.

This debate is like many others, endless. There are always going to be two sides arguing for it and against it. The points made here are focused on marijuana's medical properties and hopefully can help people decide if they want to choose it as an option or not.

CHAPTER SIXTEEN

MARIJUANA-THE DRUG

Marijuana as a drug is known to possess many attributes that can either be harmful or beneficial depending on the use. It is the most commonly used drug in the United States as well as most parts of the world. The plant of cannabis contains THC (delta-9-tetrahydrocannabinol) which is a mind altering chemical. Its extracts are also used and manufactured for medicinal properties.

Marijuana's components are used in Marinol. Now people may use Marinol and consider it similar to using marijuana as a drug. But it can be said that this might not be exactly true. It contains the THC that is just one component of marijuana. And people may not be fully availing the therapeutic advantages that might come from using marijuana in its essence.

Others may argue that it is actually for the better since Marinol as a capsule is a FDA approved drug. The FDA has not yet approved the use of marijuana as a treatment in its basic form. While Marinol can be administered in controlled dosages, marijuana cannot be contained. Many of its over four hundred properties are unstudied and remain a mystery as far as healing is concerned.

As far as its addictive properties are concerned, people remain divided over them as well. Even dispelled as a myth in an earlier chapter, it cannot be definitely concluded whether it is addictive or not.

It is regularly pitched against alcohol and other high powering drugs and has known to be rendered relatively harmless as far as addiction is concerned when compared to those. Yes it can lead to psychological dependence sometimes but when it comes to addiction, it has not yet been proved to lead to that.

People usually resort to smoking tobacco laden cigarettes more than marijuana and hence can become addicted to those or even other drugs but less likely to marijuana.

While some has said that there are no withdrawals, others have found symptoms in stuies.

There are people who say that it is possible to get addicted to marijuana as a drug and its symptoms are similar to those of nicotine. Studies might have found symptoms of marijuana withdrawal in people who after smoking it for a long time were than abstaining from it.

Withdrawal effects listed were decreased appetite, sleep difficulty, and weight loss that changed across the smoking and abstinence phases. Also others such as irritation, aggression, anger, restlessness and in some extremes even hallucinations.

Then there is the issue of marijuana being a 'Gateway drug'. This means that marijuana may not itself be harmful as much but can pave the way for harder drugs like cocaine and heroin.

While some researchers oppose the link between marijuana and other drugs, many believe that it is in fact the reason why many youngsters go on to doing hardcore drugs. Marijuana typically comes first because it is more available. Patters have shown that increases in the likelihood of cocaine and heroin use and drug dependence are also apparent for those who initiate use of marijuana at any later age.

Marijuana as a drug has mainly been a point of discussion when it comes to the young generation. Teenagers and adults between the ages of twenty-one to twenty-five are more likely to indulge in recreational use of marijuana rather than medical. Some might even use medical marijuana as habitual fun.

State laws have definitely been harder on the youth and even leading to a decline, but it doesn't negate the fact that marijuana is still legal in twenty three states and many countries as well. Than can lead many of the youngsters to gain easy access to marijuana smoking as a recreational activity more than a medicinal herb.

Looking at marijuana as a drug raises another very important question, which is that should marijuana be a used as a medical option or not?

The benefits of medical marijuana are numerous and clearly effective as well. Yet experts and physicians seem divided over this. However it is important to know that despite their contradicting views, they all seem to agree on one aspect: that marijuana is and can be used as a medicine for various purposes.

It's not about if marijuana is better or worse than other medication available. It comes down to personal choice in the end. For many medical conditions, there are a number of different medications available, some of which work better in some patients and some which work better in others.

Having the maximum number of effective medications available allows physicians to deliver the best possible medical care to individual patients.

CHAPTER SEVENTEEN

LONG TERM AND SHORT TERM EFFECTS OF MARIJUANA

Before taking any kind of medicine, it is important to be completely aware of all the possible side effects of that particular medicine. Similarly, when trying marijuana, it is also necessary that one is familiar with all the outcomes that can affect the health negatively.

The side effects of marijuana are discussed in detail in another chapter later. Here I am focusing on more of the mental effects that marijuana can have on people.

<u>Short Term</u>

When a person is taking marijuana by smoking it, these effects are more likely to present themselves. THC passes from the lungs to the bloodstream quickly when it's being inhaled. The chemicals are than carried to parts of the body and organs such as brain, etc.

The process of absorption by the body can be long or occur quickly depending on whether the person has eaten recently or not. It might take up to thirty minutes or an hour.

The effects are:

- ❖ Alteration in senses (for example, seeing brighter colors or hallucinations)
- ❖ Confusion, such as a varying sense of time.
- ❖ Mood Swings
- ❖ Impaired coordination and body movement
- ❖ Difficulty with thinking and problem solving
- ❖ Impaired memory

Long term effects have much to do with slowing of the brain development. If marijuana is being consumed over long periods of time, the brain might experience impaired function in being able to establish connection with the body properly.

Thus leading to these long term effects:

- ❖ Amnesia

- ❖ Loss of intelligence quotient

- ❖ Anxiety

- ❖ Psychosis (Severe mental disorders)

- ❖ Addiction

Although experts have been saying that the side effects of marijuana are usually mild. But that is totally dependent on its usage. If it's being consumed frequently and over a long span of time, than its effects might be lasting. Sometimes even permanent. Other than mental effects it can have damaging physical effects too. Such as difficulty in breathing, trouble in conceiving and heart rate problems. Mental toll can be seen through excessive paranoia, hallucinations and schizophrenia.

It has also been linked to depression and suicidal tendencies.

Marijuana extracts have recently been doing the rounds. This is when THC-rich resins are extracted from marijuana plants and used for rapid effectiveness. This practice is known as dabbing. Some forms of these extracts include:

- ❖ Hash oil in liquid form

- ❖ Wax that is basically a texture similar to lip balm

❖ Shatter which is a hard, amber-colored solid

These extracts are known to carry an extremely high volume of THC. The use of these extracts has sent some users to the hospital with considerable damage. For people who make this at home, the process itself can be damaging. There have been reports of fires and explosions as a light fire is used in the extracting.

Another one of marijuana's effect is the way it can impact on the quality of life. In long term, a few people have reported that marijuana has, given them lower life satisfaction, poorer mental health, poorer physical health and more relationship problems It has also been assessed that marijuana is linked to falling academic and career success. It is cited as a reason for rising school dropouts and is also linked to more job absences, accidents, and injuries.

CHAPTER EIGHTEEN

SOME HEALTH BENEFITS OF MARIJUANA

This chapter lists and analyzes the twenty-three health benefits that have been listed by major studies and have been published. The book has talked about all the health benefits and issues that come with using medical marijuana. Here, they are summarized and put together for an easy assessment.

The benefits are:

It can be used for treating Glaucoma.

Glaucoma is an eye disease that results in increased pressure in the eyeball, damage to the optic nerve and can ultimately cause loss of sight. The effects of the drug may slow the progression of the disease, preventing blindness.

It may help with the reversal of tobacco effects and actually improve lung health.

According to a study by AMA, marijuana smoking is not related to lung diseases; in fact it can increase lung capacity. Researchers examining risk factors of heart disease tested the lung function of over five thousand young adults over the course of twenty years. Tobacco smokers were losing lung function over time, but marijuana users actually showed an increase in lung capacity.

On a side note, it's been said that it could be possible that the increased lung capacity maybe due to taking deep breaths while inhaling the drug and not from a therapeutic chemical in the drug.

It helps control epileptic seizures.

A study in 2003 showed the results that it helped with the control of epilepsy. Robert J. DeLorenzo, of Virginia Commonwealth University, gave marijuana extract and synthetic marijuana to epileptic rats. The drugs were able to stop the seizures in rats for about ten hours. Cannabinoids and tetrahydrocannabinol (THC) control seizures by binding with the brain cells responsible for controlling excitement and regulating relaxation.

The findings were published in the Journal of Pharmacology and Experimental Therapeutics.

It also reduced the symptoms of a severe seizure disorder called the Dravet's Syndrome.

Dravet Syndrome causes seizures and severe developmental delays. And according to a documentary film called 'Weed' marijuana is working effectively to treat the seizures. A girl was treated by a marijuana strain, high in cannabidiol and low in THC. The film shows that since the drug was administered, her seizures decreased from three hundred a week to just one every seven days. Forty other children in the state are using the same strain of marijuana to treat their seizures, and it seems to be working.

The doctors who recommended this treatment state that the cannabidiol in the plant interacts with the brain cells to subdue the excessive activity in the brain that causes these seizures. The Drug Enforcement agency however doesn't endorse marijuana as a treatment for Dravet or other seizure disorders.

It stops cancer cell growth.

As stated previously also, cannabidiol is known to halt cancer cell growth. Cannabidiol stops cancer by turning off a gene called Id-1. A study, published in the journal Molecular Cancer Therapeutics, found that out. Cancer cells make more copies of this gene than non-cancerous cells, and it helps them spread through the body.

But after being treated with cannabidiol, the spreading stopped or in some cases slowed down.

If taken in properly, over small periods of time, it may even reduce anxiety.

Yes, quite the opposite belief. A study in Harvard Medical School discovered that when it is taken properly, it causes relaxation and act as a sedative. It becomes the cause of anxiety only when it is taken frequently for long periods of time.

THC is known to slow progress of Alzheimer's.

A 2006 study, published in the journal Molecular Pharmaceutics, found that THC slows down the formation of amyloid plaques by blocking the enzyme in the brain that is responsible for making them. These plaques are what kill brain cells and cause Alzheimer's.

Treatment for Multiple Sclerosis (MS)

It works in easing the pain in muscles by binding itself to nerve muscles.

It also helps with other muscles spasms as well.

A research found that a person suffering from diaphragm spasms was using marijuana to treat them. It seemed to work when other, more powerful drugs did not.

It lessens side effects from Hepatitis C and increases the effectiveness of the treatment.

Treatment for hepatitis C infection is hard and negative side effects include fatigue, nausea, muscle aches, loss of appetite, and depression. They may last for months. Many people aren't able to finish their treatment course because of the side effects.

A 2006 study in the European Journal of Gastroenterology and Hepatology found that eighty-six percent of patients using marijuana successfully completed their Hep C treatment while only thirty percent of non-smokers completed theirs. This could have been possible because of the marijuana which helped lessened the treatments side effects.

Marijuana also seems to improve the treatment's effectiveness: Fifty four percent of hep C patients smoking marijuana got their viral levels low, in comparison to only eight percent of nonsmokers.

It treats inflammatory bowel disease.

It helps with diseases such as ulcers by blocking the bacteria and binding intestinal cells together tightly.

It helps with arthritis.

It was observed that Sativax was able to relieve discomfort in arthritis patients. A university of Nottingham study discovered that when rheumatology departments gave their patients the medicine carrying cannibinoids. They experienced a significant reduction in pain and better quality of sleep.

It helps increase metabolic function.

A study published in the American Journal of Medicine on April of last year, suggested that marijuana smokers have faster metabolism than the average person. The study analyzed data from over four thousand users, and it came to the conclusion that their reaction to sugars is also different than that of non-smokers. Their body has a healthier response to sugars.

It improves the symptoms of Lupus.

Lupus is an autoimmune disorder known as the Systemic Lupus Ertyhematosus, which is when the body starts attacking itself for any unknown reason. Some chemicals in marijuana seem to have a calming effect on the immune system, which could be how it helps deal with symptoms of Lupus.

It helps with Crohn's disease.

This is an inflammatory bowel disease that results in diarrohea, vomiting and stomach pains. Marijuana helps in subsiding those and many patients have seen recovery after using it.

Soothes tremors in Parkinson's disease.

A research from Israel showed that smoking marijuana could lead to reduction of pain and tremors in patients of Parkinson's. It led to improved sleep as well. What was surprising was the remarkable improvement in coordination and movement was among patients.

Medical marijuana is legal in Israel, and a lot of research into the medical uses of cannabis is done there. The Israeli government supports it.

It is known to be helpful with PTSD symptoms.

Recently the Department of Health and Human Services signed off on a proposal to study marijuana's potential as part of treatment for veterans with post-traumatic stress disorder.

Marijuana is approved to treat PTSD in some states already. In New Mexico, PTSD is the primary reason for people to secure a license for medical marijuana, but this is the first time the U.S. government has approved a proposal that is incorporating smoked or vaporized marijuana as a treatment.

Its components are known to be regulating the fear and anxiety in the body.

It might protect the brain after a stroke.

Research has led to conclusions being made that it can protect the brain after a stroke or concussions by reducing the size of the affected areas.

It might even protect from trauma.

It can help reduce nightmares.

In patients of PTSD, it can help by interrupting REM sleep.

Marijuana is safer than alcohol.

It helps with chemotherapy.

Marijuana helps stimulate brain function and increases creativity levels as well.

These are some of the benefits that were observed and summarized to give the people an idea of what medical marijuana is really about.

CHAPTER NINETEEN

MEDICAL MARIJUANA AND STATE LAWS

The United States has not yet legalized use, possession, sale, cultivation, and transportation of cannabis (marijuana) in the United States under federal law is but the federal government has announced that if a state wants to pass a law to decriminalize cannabis for recreational or medical use they can do that. But that is only if they have a regulatory system monitoring the use of cannabis.

The Controlled Substances Act of 1970 classifies marijuana is classifies as a Schedule I substance, the highest classification under the legislation. This means that the substance has been claimed by the U.S. federal government to have both high abuse potential and no established medical use.

However despite hindrances in Federal law there are twenty three states now that have legalized the use of marijuana. Many of those have only allowed it for medical use.

Those twenty-three states are:

1. Alabama
2. Arizona
3. California
4. Colorado
5. Connecticut
6. DC
7. Delaware
8. Hawaii
9. Illinois
10. Maine
11. Maryland
12. Massachusetts
13. Michigan
14. Montana
15. Minnesota
16. Nevada
17. New Hampshire

18. New Jersey

19. New York

20. New Mexico

21. Oregon

22. Rhode Island

23. Vermont

The use of both recreational and medicinal marijuana has been completely legalized in the states of Colorado, Washington, Alaska and Oregon. The cities of both Portland and South Portland in Maine also fully legalized marijuana for both medical and recreational use. The District of Columbia has legalized recreational and medical marijuana, but Congress currently blocks recreational commercial sale for now. Other twelve states have both medical marijuana and decriminalization laws. Ten states, including Guam and Puerto Rico have legalized only medical marijuana. The Virgin Islands along with a couple of others states also just decriminalized their possession laws.

The remaining twenty-two states and two other inhabited territories contain the law that marijuana is illegal, an offensive felony, or a misdemeanor.

State wise every law differs. When it comes to medical marijuana many realize its potential as a treatment drug and thus are now easing their laws around it. But there are some which still hold the idea that it is a negative influence on the society especially on the youth.

California became the first in all of the states to legalize medical marijuana when the Proposition 215 was passed. And since then twenty-two others have followed suit.

A total of these states, along with the District of Columbia and Guam now allow for comprehensive public medical marijuana and cannabis programs. There were recent efforts made towards the legalization cause, as a result of those, approvals in seventeen states came for the use of strains of low THC and high cannabidiol' products. These were to be used for medical reasons only if the situation demanded.

These efforts were a result of programs that allowed:

❖ Protection from prosecution and criminal penalties for using marijuana as a medicine.

❖ Access to marijuana through freely; through home cultivation, dispensaries or some other system that is likely to be implemented.

❖ It allows for a variety of strains to be readily available, including those more than "low THC".

❖ It allows both smoking and vaporization of any kind of marijuana products, plant material or extracts.

The Institute of Medicine ratified California's Prop 215 by agreeing with the hypothesis that marijuana was indeed helpful with chronic diseases such as MS and cancer, and carried therapeutic value. They also agreed that the psychological effects that are induced by high potency marijuana smoking marred its therapeutic benefits.

State vs. Federal

At the federal level, marijuana has remained classified as a Schedule I substance under the Controlled Substances Act, as said earlier, the Schedule I substances are considered to have a high potential for dependency and no accepted medical use. This makes distribution of marijuana a federal offense.

In October of 2009, the Obama Administration took initiative to try and relax these laws a bit. They sent a memo to federal prosecutors encouraging them to not prosecute people who are found distributing marijuana for medical purposes in accordance with state law.

In August 2013, the U.S. Department of Justice (USDOJ) came up an announcement regarding an update to their marijuana enforcement policy. The statement contained that while marijuana remains illegal on a federal level, the USDOJ will not challenge the states own local drug enforcement laws if it allowed marijuana use. In states like Colorado, the Justice department asked for stronger enforcement and agreed upon just monitoring the states laws. However the department admitted that it does reserve the right to challenge and regulate the states' policy at any time they feel necessary.

Voters in Arizona and the District of Columbia passed initiatives to allow for medical use but to little avail as they were overturned. In 1998, voters in the District of Columbia passed Initiative 59 that promoted the use of medical marijuana. But the Congress blocked the initiative and stopped it from becoming law. However in 2009, Congress reversed its previous decision and allowed the initiative to become law. Before the passing of Proposition 203 in 2010, the Arizona voters originally had passed ballot. The initiative gave permission to the doctors to approve prescriptions for marijuana. This was in contradiction with the state law. Marijuana is a Schedule I substance, hence federal law does not allow it to be prescribed, and that invalidated the ballot.

Medical marijuana cannot be prescribed officially. The doctors may call the prescriptions as a recommendation or a referral, because of the prohibition that the federal law places on this.

States with medical marijuana laws are able to provide protection against marijuana possession arrests. They generally have some form of patient registry, and that may provide some relief and exemption from prosecution for possession of a certain amount of marijuana for personal medicinal use. Most states where it is legal have even stated the amount of marijuana in weight that is okay to keep with oneself at a time.

This is one way where it can be regulated and monitored. Some of the most common policy questions raised regarding medical marijuana are about its regulation, recommendation, dispensing, and registration of approved patients.

Some states and localities that are without dispensary regulation have been experiencing a boost in new businesses. They hope of getting approved before presumably stricter regulations are enforced. Medical marijuana dispensaries and cultivators are often termed to as caregivers.

Even they may have to adhere to limitations as to giving out a certain amount of extracts and products to one patient.

CHAPTER TWENTY

10 PHARMACEUTICAL DRUGS WITH CANNABIS

There are several pharmaceutical drugs that have been developed which carry similar chemicals or properties as those that are present in the cannabis plant. This process started after research started highlighting all the positives that were derived from marijuana in medicine.

Some researchers have furthered their research by using their understanding of the ways that the brain processes and utilizes the cannabinoids to develop drugs. These drugs follow the same pattern but carry different properties and effects than those of marijuana's.

A list of those pharmaceutical drugs based on marijuana is given below. All details are included for the benefit of the people who might consider choosing these drugs. Along with their names, manufacturing companies, and cannabis properties, their medical uses that have been suggested by experts, and approval status are also given.

1. Sativex (directly contains Marijuana chemicals)

It is a mouth spray whose compounds are derived from extracts of the cannabis plant. It contains two cannabinoids: THC and CBD.

It enables the treatment of neuropathic pain and spasms in patients with Multiple Sclerosis. It can provide relief to adult patients with advanced cancer. It is known to help those patients that may experience different levels of pain.

It was approved and launched in the markets of United Kingdom on June 21, 2010, making it the first ever cannabis containing prescription medicine found globally.

In Spain on July 28, 2010, it was approved to treat spasticity caused by multiple sclerosis.

In Canada and many European countries such as Austria, Germany, Italy and Sweden it was approved in the period from 2010 to 2011. Switzerland also gave it the stamp of approval in 2013.

In the US, however the process is ongoing. Clinical trials started in late 2006 for pain treatment in cancer patients.

In 2011, the US granted a patent for Sativex use in cancer pain. However as of 2014, Sativex is still in development for treatment of pain within patients suffering from cancer.

GW Pharmaceuticals along with Otsuka Pharmaceutical started an Investigational New Drug application in the United States for treatment of spasms in Multiple Sclerosis.

However in January 2015, after a year since it started in August 2014, results could not be produced as hoped. There are still two additional Phase 3 trials in progress currently.

2. Marinol

It is manufactured by Unimed Pharmaceuticals, which is Solvay Pharmaceuticals' subsidiary.

It can be used for the treatment of vomiting and nausea in patients who have cancer. It is also found to be an appetite stimulant for AIDS patients as well and known to ease neuropathic pain in multiple sclerosis patients.

The FDA approved it in United States as a drug for appetite stimulation and for nausea in in 1992 and 1985 respectively. It was moved to a Schedule III (less potential for abuse and medical acceptance) drug, effective in July 2, 1999. It was also approved in Denmark for MS in September 2003.

It then got its approval in Canada for anorexia that is found in AIDS patients. It was also approved for treating vomiting and nausea that is caused by cancer chemotherapy in 1988.

The rest are all drugs that carry chemical properties similar to those found in Marijuana but are not exactly from the plant.

3. Nabilone / Cesamet

It is made by Valeant Pharmaceuticals.

It is suggested for the treatment of nausea and vomiting in patients undergoing cancer treatment.

It was originally approved by the FDA as a proper drug in the United States in 1985, but was subsequently removed from the market. It was then re-launched by the FDA on May 15, 2006 and could be found in US pharmacies within a couple of months.

It got approval in United Kingdom and Australia in 1982, Canada in 1981, and Mexico in 2007.

In May 2006, the FDA called for safety labeling in nabilone to warn people about precautions related to its use, such as the potential to affect the mental state of a patient.

Valeant announced in February 2007, that it would be submitting an Investigational New Drug application to test Cesamet as a treatment for chemotherapy induced pain.

4. Dexanabinol

Manufactured by Solvay Pharmaceuticals, it is a drug that can act as a neuro-protective agent for use after cardiac surgery. It can help with the recovery of memory and other brain functions following Traumatic Brain Injury. There is also a possibility of its future use as an anti-cancer drug. It is not approved for use as of Nov. 11, 2013.

A clinical trial with more than eight hundred patients was completed in December 2004. It was revealed that the drug had failed to show any significant improvement in the late stage of the trial.

5. CT-3

It is made by Indevus Pharmaceuticals. It could be utilized as a potential treatment for spasticity and pain in patients suffering from MS. It may also help relieve pain from arthritis. It has not been approved for use as of Nov. 11, 2013.

It completed Phase I clinical trials as of July 2002.Another study started in May 2002, Germany. This was to test its pain relieving properties in patients who experienced neuropathic pain.

6. Cannabinor

It is known to be anti-inflammatory. It can also be used as a treatment for chronic pain focusing especially on nerve pain.

It also helps with control of bladder. It cannot be used outside of laboratory research.

In the UK, trials began towards the end of 2006. In January 2007, it was reported that in those trials, cannabinor had failed to reach its goal of reducing induced pain through capsaicin. The drug however was found to be safe.

7. HU 308

It is manufactured by Pharmos. It is can used in the treatment of hypertension and is also anti-inflammatory. Again, this has also not been approved for use outside of laboratory research as of November 11, 2013. It did demonstrate efficacy in some laboratory studies.

8. HU 331

Cayman Chemicals makes this drug. It can be helpful with treatment of memory and weight loss. Also stimulates appetite, prevents neuro-degeneration and provides tumor surveillance. It is known to be useful with pain and inflammation relief as well. It has not been approved for use apart from laboratory research as of 2013.

Cayman Chemical says that currently no studies were taking place. However, the HU 331 could be purchased through research institutions. The other two drugs on the list only function in similar ways but have no actual similarity with marijuana.

9. Rimonabant

10. Taranabant

The FDA does not approve both of them. The purpose of giving all such details about these drugs was to familiarize people with medicines that are associated with marijuana in order to give them a better understanding of its properties and uses.

CHAPTER TWENTY ONE

MEDICAL OPINION ON MARIJUANA

After reading so much about marijuana and its uses in medicine, one might actually be interested to know what some doctors and experts have to say about medical marijuana.

These are some statements made by Surgeon Generals that are appointed by the President and confirmed by the Senate. Recently, Dr. Vivek Murthy serving from 2014 has also made a statement regarding it,

He stated that he was interested in exploring further possibilities. He said that interested in seeing what scientific research showed about the efficiency of marijuana. He admitted to looking through preliminary data which showed certain medical conditions and symptoms could be helped by the use of that marijuana. He has not clearly expressed as to which side of the yes or no debate he is on, but there are others who express their views against it and for its use.

M. Joycelyn Elders serving from 1993 to 1994 and appointed by President Clinton have expressed favorable views for the use of medical marijuana. She stated that the evidence of the benefits of marijuana is very much there. It can indeed relieve certain types of pain and vomiting. It is also a safe drug, significantly less toxic than many of the drugs that physicians mostly prescribe.

Other than that there are many physicians who advocate its use while others are of the opinion that it should be restricted.

All the ones working for its legalization cite reasons based on marijuana's ability to ease pain, stop vomiting, and help patients with AIDS and cancer. They do believe that it comes with its harm but so does every other thing.

If used in the right quantity and with proper precaution it can be quite beneficial. Many physicians who are against its uses, lists all the negative aspects of it. First and foremost it involves smoking.

Then it can spur addiction. If someone like absolutely wants to use it, they can consider it in its drug form, like Marinol.

A physician summed up all his colleagues similar views in an article against the use of medical marijuana. He wrote that medical marijuana studies had raised more questions than they answered. There were too many harmful consequences and unknown variables that presented risks.

Marijuana's use as a prescription drug was in violation of safety protocols and does not match the standard of drugs. Most physicians will not prescribe a drug that has not been put thorough patient safety testing and trials. The last choice lies with the patients eventually. They must choose their own treatment in light of credible evidence.

He said that he, along with many other physicians chose not to prescribe marijuana for long term and critical illnesses based upon this evidence. It would be ethical to prescribe a medication that can cause addiction from over use and additional harm to health.

This reflects most of the doctors' view that are not in favor of it. Marijuana has been compared to FDA approved drugs and the death rate from both is analyzed as to show how marijuana users fare when compared to the other drug users. And the results were surprising. The death count from marijuana was approximately under three hundred, while from other drugs it went on to over eleven thousand.

Medical opinion has been discussed but what does the public have to say about it? Public opinion on medical marijuana is also varied but it is tilting increasingly in favor of it.

A narrow majority, 53% of Americans say the drug should be made legal, compared with 44% who want it to be illegal. Opinions have undergone significant changes since 1969, when the first questions regarding marijuana legalization were raised. At the time, only twelve percent people were in of the view that marijuana use should be legalized. Much of the change in opinion has occurred over the past five to ten years. Support rose eleven points between 2010 and 2013 Seven in ten Americans, almost 69%, are of the opinion that alcohol is more damaging to a person's health than marijuana. While 15% pick marijuana as worse.

If marijuana became as widely available as alcohol, 63% still believe alcohol would be more damaging to society. Even President Obama agreed that alcohol is more harmful than marijuana. Nearly half of Americans say they have tried marijuana. About 12% have been reported as using it in the past year. The 2012 National Survey on Drug Use and Health says it is the most commonly used illegal drug in the U.S.

There are some who still remain bothered by it and shy away from its use. It has garnered this increased support from the youth, democrats and Independents, as well as liberals.

Although independents and Democrats have always been more likely than Republicans to support legalization of marijuana, but over the past forty years, the gap between their views on this issue has increased substantially. Recently the democrats and independents are known to show more inclination towards favoring marijuana legalization and agree that it should be made legal. This has been a major change in their opinion compared to ten years before.

The views of Republicans are practically unchanged. Many analysts have even said that the Obama administration has views in support of legalization as well. Almost half of both Democrats and independents now support the legalization of marijuana with their respective percentages being 48% and 49%. Where else, 24% of Republicans support legalization now, similar to the 26% who favored this more than a decade ago. 71% of Republicans, along 77% of conservative Republicans, are strictly in opposition of the legalization of marijuana

There are substantial demographic differences in opinions about the legalization of marijuana. A majority of the people younger than thirty thinks that the use of marijuana should be made legal. There are gender based demographic differences as well. While men are evenly divided over whether the use of marijuana should be legal, most women oppose legalization.

People residing in states where medical marijuana laws already have been passed are more likely to support marijuana's legalization than those living in other states where it is not legal. Those who have tried marijuana are also more likely to campaign for the legalization of marijuana, compared to those who have not tried it.

CHAPTER TWENTY TWO

WHO SHOULDN'T USE MARIJUANA?

Medical marijuana isn't recommended for anyone under the age of 18 years of age. That is currently under review for children with epilepsy, cancer and other chronic illnesses. Many parents are seeking out cannabis resources for their children because the FDA approved medications aren't helping their children and marijuana may just be their answer. At this time, doctors are not allowed to prescribe medical marijuana for children under the age of 18. Thus, children should avoid its use. Since this is very similar to the decision to drink strong alcohol, its common sense under general law that children should be excluded unless supervised by parents who are caring for children. This refers to children that can potentially find therapeutic help from the use of marijuana should the laws be changed to allow them to benefit from its use to have access to a prescription specific to their illness.

Caution should be used when prescribing marijuana to anyone with a history of psychosis. As mentioned previously, numerous cases of anxiety, panic attacks and psychotic issues with patients having a history of these mental health problems have been documented. Thus, if you do suffer from any of the ailments described, it's vital to seek the help of your general practitioner to find out if marijuana is suitable for your use for medical purposes.

Pregnant women should not use marijuana. It's been proven that smoking causes damage to a fetus. Also, there is some indication that a fetus can be harmed by the mothers' use of marijuana in any form. Thus using marijuana in edibles should also be avoided.

Growing Your Own Marijuana

You should always be aware that there would be legal restrictions in whatever area of the world you live in and that you need to abide by those restrictions. This will limit the amount of plants that you can have. There are reports that people have had plants stolen at the height of the harvest time, and since this is common, it's a good idea to grow your plants in an area where you can control this. A private garden that is closed off is preferable. If you want to grow your plants indoors and use an artificial lighting system to produce the seasons that the plant needs to mature, lights can be purchased which can be mounted above the plants. You must study the growing season. In nature, the plants would expect the same seasons to occur every year, though in a false environment, you can bring plants on quite quickly.

Seeds can be sewn on blotting paper on a windowsill that will give the seeds adequate light. The blotting paper should be placed over a small saucer of water, just like you would with cress seeds. Once the plants have started to show small roots, they can be moved to small pots, using a rich soil that gives them sufficient drainage during the time that they develop their root system. At this stage, they are still small enough to keep on a windowsill so that they gain sufficient natural light.

If you are going to grow your plants outside, this takes place after you have moved the plant from the small pot to a larger one. Take the plant outside in the sunshine, but bring it in at night to protect it from any coldness. Gradually transplant the plants into the ground, after they have weathered off for a while and are accustomed to the outside air. This is suitable in areas with good sunshine, as they need this sunshine to grow to their full potential. Some people hide their plants under wooded areas, though this isn't really suitable, since they do not get enough sunlight and the acid from the conifers within the woodland may actually spoil the crop.

You could alternatively use a cold frame until the plants are strong enough to be planted in their permanent patch. If you subject a plant to bad weather too early on in its growth, it will stem full growth of the plant. This is a hot climate plant. Thus, if you live in an area that cannot produce that temperature that the plant needs, heat lamps indoors make a good alternative. If you decide to use this indoor method, it's wise to read up fully on the times of using the lights, rather than to use them indiscriminately. Each grower has their own secret additives for soils and talking with other growers will help you to increase your efficiency to grow your own crop.

As stated in the beginning of this section, do check with the law what is legal for you to grow. Although medical marijuana may be the norm in the state where you live, there may still be restrictions as to how many plants you can grow and fines for people found to be exceeding this, since they may be considered to be potential dealers. Also be aware that hydroponics, or growing under lamps, will cost rather a lot in electricity consumption so if you are in rented property and do not pay for the electric supply, it may be a good idea to clear this with the owner.

Remember that it is the female plant that gives the heads that are the part of the plant that is consumed. Do talk to other growers about their supplies of seeds and the ratio they use of male/female plants. Too many males and the females can lose their potency. Get the mix wrong, and your crop may be useless.

Thus, if you have a green thumb and are able to grow your own, within the boundaries of the law, then this is probably the best source you can have because you will know that the marijuana that you produce is pure and has not been mixed with other contaminants while en route to your location.

If you don't have the patience for gardening or looking after your own crop, try to find out from your doctor or marijuana clinic where you can get organically grown marijuana.

Learn to take your crop at the right time from other growers. Use their experience to help you to decide the best time. There are those that swear by the full moon being a good time to take in the crop, though this is only speculation and really depends upon where you are growing it and what your climate is like. The full moon connection may simply be a grower's superstition that works for him/her.

CONCLUSION

There has been a great deal of confusion for many years about the benefits of marijuana due to several books, campaigns and reports offering biased or confusing information. Some sources used by readers to find out information may not even be that accurate and some may give wrongful information. Many states have taken the bold step to legalize medical marijuana; other states are still lagging behind. Some states have even legalized the use of marijuana for recreational purposes. It is hoped that this book has given you unbiased information needed to help you make an informed decision about your own medical care. Remember to always consult professionals who will know the types of plant that can help with your particular illness. The book outlines the law in different parts of the world; it shows you the states that have legalized the use of marijuana and gives information on the illnesses that marijuana is able to help with.

It should also be noted by readers that the book is neither suggesting nor condemning the use of marijuana but is based on medical information available to everyone. This has been compiled in an easy to read format so that all the information needed by a potential marijuana user is in one place, thus making answers to their questions easier to find. There is a great deal of controversy worldwide about the use of marijuana. Being informed as to its history, its use and its potential beneficial effects helps you to make better decisions about whether this is a natural herb that can help you in the healing process, or at least make your life a little easier along the way. It has been well researched and covers the topic comprehensively, thus helping you in your search for information applicable to you.

www.ingramcontent.com/pod-product-compliance
Lightning Source LLC
Chambersburg PA
CBHW062007280526
45787CB00005B/2009